Arthritis Without Pain

The Miracle of TNF Blockers

Arthritis Without Pain is directed to patients with rheumatoid arthritis and related disorders. The book is not intended to provide personal medical advice and should not be used as an alternative to appropriate medical care. The reader should always consult his/her personal physician before undergoing any medical therapy or changes in medical therapy. Furthermore, if the reader encounters information in this book that differs from advice given by a physician, he/she should discuss it with the physician.

The authors have made every effort to ensure that the information presented here is accurate as of the date of publication. However, in light of ongoing research and the constant flow of information, it is possible that new findings may invalidate data or facts presented in this book. In addition, dose schedules are being continually revised and new side effects recognized. The authors, editor, reviewers, publisher and distributors of this book are not liable for any inadvertent errors or misinterpretation or misuse of the information printed in this book; and make no representation, express or implied, that the drug dosages, regimens, side effects and recommendations discussed in this book are correct. For these reasons, the reader is strongly urged to consult his/her physician and the drug manufacturer's printed instructions before taking any medication.

Dr. Scott J. Zashin has been a paid consultant and/or speaker for the companies whose products are listed in this book.

The authors do not endorse any company or product mentioned in this book. When the authors were aware of a trademarked product or drug name, the trademark is noted. The authors, editor and publishers are not responsible for inadvertent omission of trademarks. The trademarks and registered trademarks used throughout the text to identify brand names of drugs and products are the property of their respective trademark holders.

The names of the people with arthritis who are quoted or mentioned in this book have been changed to protect their privacy. All are current or former patients of Dr. Zashin.

ISBN 0-9754060-0-0

Produced in the United States of America

Revised July 2004

Contents

Acknowledgments

I gratefully acknowledge the courage and cooperation of the many patients whose stories and clinical successes inspired me to write this book. I especially want to thank the patients[1] who shared their experiences, and allowed us to write about them.

I also acknowledge my nurses and professional staff for the concern and caring they show all of our patients, and for their support of and enthusiasm for this project. My heartfelt thanks go to Sharon Baker, R.N.; Katie Berkstresser; Suzanne Booth, R.N.; Terry Crabtree, L.V.N.; Chrissy Dickey, M.L.T., M.R.T.; Laura Gomez, R.N.; Terri Groom; Suzanne Kelly, R.N.; Kristin Knight; Norma Kolski, P.B.T., N.C.T.; Sarah Merrifield, R.N.; Penny Allen, M.L.T.; Maureen Rump, R.N.; and Vickie Skillestad, R.N.

Finally, I am grateful to John Cush, M.D., David Karp, M.D., Ph.D. and Salahuddin Kazi, M.D. for their insights and input in reviewing the manuscript; to Laura Gomez, R.N., for the book's title; and to Amy Ray and Kay Martin for proofreading.

— Scott J. Zashin, M.D.

---

1 Patients' names have been changed throughout the book to protect their privacy.

About the Authors

Scott J. Zashin, M.D., is a clinical assistant professor at the University of Texas Southwestern Medical School, Division of Rheumatology, in Dallas, Texas, as well as an attending physician at Presbyterian Hospitals of Dallas and Plano. He is a fellow of the American College of Physicians and the American College of Rheumatology and a member of the American Medical Association.

A native of Short Hills, New Jersey, Dr. Zashin earned his medical and undergraduate degrees from Dartmouth College. He continued his medical training in Dallas at Parkland Hospital and the University of Texas Southwestern Medical School. Dr. Zashin is board-certified in both internal medicine and rheumatology.

Dr. Zashin has published many articles about arthritis, and is a sought-after speaker on numerous topics relating to both traditional and alternative arthritis treatments. He is presently a member of the speaker's bureaus for several pharmaceutical companies, including Abbott Laboratories and Wyeth-Ayerst. He has conducted clinical studies for Amgen and Merck. Dr. Zashin is currently president of the North Texas Chapter of the Lupus Foundation, and for the past eight years, has been recognized as an outstanding physician in the Woodward White publication, *Best Doctors of America — Central Region*.

Dr. Zashin lives in Dallas with his wife, Angela, and two daughters.

M. Laurette Hesser has worked with patients, physicians and clinicians for two decades to create educational programs and publications that promote understanding and facilitate delivery of care. A marketing and corporate communications consultant with a special interest in healthcare issues, Ms. Hesser has developed programs and materials for many organizations, including Advanced Neuromodulation Systems, CerebroVascular Advances, Novation, Quest Medical, Synthes (USA) and Urologix, as well as ExxonMobil, IBM, Nortel, Southern Methodist University, The City of Irving (Texas) and CEC Entertainment. A native of Pennsylvania, she earned a B.S. degree in marketing from Penn State. Ms. Hesser resides in Dallas with her husband, Tom.

Preface

I would never have imagined that a freshman writing course I reluctantly enrolled in 27 years ago would one day be linked to my interest in writing this book.

In 1977, I was a freshman at Dartmouth College, enrolled in a liberal arts curriculum. All freshman were required to take a writing course, and the one that caught my interest dealt with cancer. The course instructor was a graduate student. I had heard that grad students did not teach courses at Dartmouth, and approached the instructor, Steve Gillis, about it. He convinced me that the course would be worth my while.

Indeed it was. Dr. Gillis (he subsequently completed his Ph.D.) allowed me to work in a research lab with Paul Baker, Ph.D., under the direction of Kendall Smith, M.D. The opportunity to work with these investigators was a rewarding experience. These scientists were later credited with the purification of a substance called interleukin-2 (IL-2), which has become an important drug in the fight against cancer and HIV.

Although IL-2 would not prove helpful for rheumatoid arthritis, the Dartmouth connection would. Dr. Gillis left Dartmouth and later started a drug company called Immunex — the company that originally developed Enbrel®, one of the TNF-blocking drugs that are the focus of this book. (Immunex was acquired by Amgen in July 2002.) Although Dr. Gillis did not participate in this book, our chance meeting at Dartmouth followed decades later by a parallel interest in a remarkable drug therapy is a wonderful coincidence.

Scott J. Zashin, M.D.
Dallas, Texas
May 8, 2004

This book is dedicated to my loving family — Angela, Sarah and Allison — as well as my parents, Walter and Carol, and my brother, Mark, who would skip his own soccer practices at The Pingry School to watch the Millburn games.

CHAPTER 1

——

Lives Renewed

"A miracle."

That was Julie Barton's first thought as she awoke on Valentine's Day 2000. For seven years, morning had become a series of slow, painful rituals as she gently coaxed her stiff joints to limber up just enough to get out of bed. As the 52-year-old floral designer stood to make her way to the bathroom, she walked on the sides of her feet, trying to avoid the tortuous sensation that she was treading on shards of hot broken glass. But this morning was different. One day after her rheumatologist, Dr. Scott Zashin, had given her a new injectable drug for rheumatoid arthritis (RA), the stiffness was noticeably less. And the pain? It was *gone*.

For Carla Mason, the transition from pain to freedom was more subtle but no less dramatic. The former international flight attendant, whose RA forced her to retire at the age of 41, had long ago learned not to get her hopes up when it came to relieving the relentless pain and inflammation in her joints. But a week after starting this new therapy for RA, her wedding band fit again. Within a month, she was back with her astronomy club and attending telescope star parties. She could now walk up the steps to the observatory. Once there, she no longer feared that the cool night air would bring on intense pain.

In the four years since starting this amazing drug treatment, Carla achieved a lifelong dream of earning a college degree, graduating with honors from the University of Texas. She is now pursuing a master's degree full-time, while working part-time as a graduate teaching assistant. She also volunteers as a tutor for a writing lab, and travels to conferences where she speaks to academicians from around the world. Rheumatoid arthritis no longer grounds Carla or her aspirations. Best of all, there are moments when she forgets completely that she has RA.

Brad Prater can't forget that he has a form of arthritis known as ankylosing spondylitis. He has lived with the disease for 25 years, and the memory of his father struggling with the same illness without the benefit of a diagnosis or viable treatment is forever etched into his mind. But Brad knows that he will fare far better than his father. This new drug therapy that he started last year is one of the first ever to get to the root of his disease. Already he is doing things at age 50 that he would not have felt well enough to do 20 years ago.

Brad now stands erect; it feels more comfortable to do so. Pain no longer limits his life. His Crohn's disease has improved, too. He feels well enough to attend the local high school's football and basketball games to see his daughter cheer. He is a regular spectator at his oldest son's soccer matches. Even his wife says he does pretty well keeping up with their four-year-old. For Brad, this therapy is one of the best things that has happened in his life. Better yet, he knows that if heredity proves unkind to his sons, this breakthrough in arthritis treatment — and the ones that will surely follow because of it — will allow his boys to be the first generation of three not to know the pain and despair of ankylosing spondylitis.

Bob Honeywell had learned to live with his arthritis over the last 15 years. The problem was the psoriasis that accompanied it. The 46-year-old sales executive traveled frequently to make presentations. He knew that customers noticed his skin condition. Bob had tried all the standard treatments, but the side effects made it difficult to continue. And none had helped the psoriasis.

In 2000, his former rheumatologist in Atlanta tracked him down in Dallas to tell him that a new therapy for RA was also yielding great results for psoriatic arthritis. Bob's new rheumatologist, Dr. Zashin, was aware of the early study results, but hesitated to recommend the medication because it was still considered experimental for psoriatic arthritis. Bob insisted that he understood the risks and wanted to try. Three days after his first injection, he had no stiffness, no soreness, no aches, and his psoriasis began to improve. So too, has his outlook on life. In the three years since he began treatment, it continues to bring Bob relief from his symptoms. For Bob, growing old is now much less of a concern. Like Julie, Carla and Brad, his life has been renewed.

The reason is a breakthrough arthritis treatment called *TNF blockers*.

CHAPTER 2

An Overview of Arthritis

Millions of people, including children, have some form of arthritis. Its tell-tale signs are pain, stiffness, and swelling in or around the joints. It is a chronic condition that can interfere with the simplest of daily activities, and is the number-one cause of painful and limited movement among adults.

More than 100 types of arthritis have been identified. Yet the cause of this destructive disorder is still not well understood. Heredity, injury, and/or environmental "insults" are thought to play a role in bringing about the joint destruction that is the hallmark of many types of arthritis. There is no cure for the structural damage from arthritis. For most types of arthritis, treatment is focused on controlling pain and inflammation.

The two most prevalent types of arthritis are osteoarthritis and rheumatoid arthritis.

OSTEOARTHRITIS: A CONDITION OF WEAR AND TEAR

Osteoarthritis (OA) is the most common form of arthritis. More than 23 million Americans have OA. Over one-third are women. The vast majority are 45 years or older. Most people believe that OA is a natural consequence of aging, but heredity and injury are equally strong risk factors.

Osteoarthritis occurs when the protective cartilage that covers the joint wears away. The joint space narrows, bone spurs form, the joint becomes inflamed, and the nerve endings become irritated.

People with osteoarthritis usually complain of joint pain after any activity involving that joint. Morning pain and stiffness are also common, but usually resolve after 15 to 30 minutes. Over time, as the cartilage continues to wear, pain often increases.

The hands, feet, knees, hips and spine (cervical spine/neck and lumbar spine/low back) are the most common areas affected by OA. Osteoarthritis of the hands often strikes the base of the thumb, at the end and middle joints. It is also common in the base of the big toe, and foot pain is worsened by tight shoes and heels. People with OA of the hips feel pain in their groin and thighs, which sometimes travels or "refers" to the knee. People with OA of the knee complain of pain and stiffness around the joint.

Osteoarthritis can severely restrict mobility and movement. Osteoarthritis of the hip and knee can cause pain with even simple weight-bearing activities, such as walking. Osteoarthritis of the hands impairs activities that require dexterity and hand strength. Pain due to OA of the spine often increases when rising from a sitting or lying position, and worsens with prolonged standing or walking.

A diagnosis of osteoarthritis is based on patient history, a physical exam, and x-rays. X-rays show narrowed joint spaces (due to loss of cartilage) and spur formation. Laboratory studies may also be performed, and results will be normal if it truly is OA. (An abnormal lab result may suggest that there is another cause of the pain, or may indicate that two types of arthritis are present.)

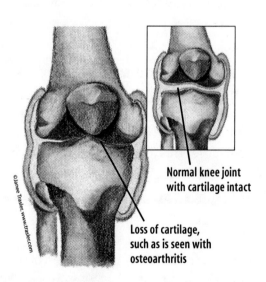

Normal knee joint with cartilage intact

Loss of cartilage, such as is seen with osteoarthritis

©Jamee Trasler, www.trasler.com

Osteoarthritis occurs when the protective cartilage that covers the joint wears away. The joint space narrows, bone spurs form, the joint becomes inflamed and the nerve endings become irritated. The result is pain, especially with use.

There is no cure for osteoarthritis. Treatment focuses on relieving pain, reducing inflammation and improving joint motion. Common medications used to treat OA include both prescription drugs and over-the-counter medications, including acetaminophen, non-steroidal anti-inflammatory drugs (NSAIDs) such as ibuprofen, and COX-2 inhibitors[2] like Celebrex®. Glucosamine is another treatment that some patients find helpful with the pain of OA, and is available over the counter. A large clinical trial at the National Institutes of Health (NIH) is underway to determine the safety and effectiveness of glucosamine in OA.

In addition to drug therapy, people with osteoarthritis are usually encouraged to exercise, which increases flexibility and builds muscle strength. Controlling body weight is another good strategy because it helps to lessen stress on weight-bearing joints. Surgery is also sometimes recommended to relieve pain in damaged joints, or to replace joints that are severely damaged.

RHEUMATOID ARTHRITIS: AN AUTOIMMUNE DISORDER THAT AFFECTS THE JOINTS

Rheumatoid arthritis (RA) affects about 1 percent of the general population. This translates to more than 2 million Americans, with a 5:2 ratio of women to men. RA strikes many people in the prime of their lives, and most often affects people in their early 30s to 60s.

Rheumatoid arthritis is a different illness than osteoarthritis. RA causes considerably more inflammation than osteoarthritis because it is an autoimmune disorder. This

---

2 NSAIDs and COX-2 inhibitors are discussed in more detail in Chapters 3 and 4.

means that the body's immune system reacts against itself. In the case of RA, the immune system destroys the joints. Inflammation results in swelling, warmth and subsequent pain in the joints. Unlike osteoarthritis, RA affects the entire body. People diagnosed with RA often complain of extreme fatigue and a general sense of malaise.

RA can range in severity from manageable to mildly disabling to completely debilitating. Early diagnosis is important in slowing the progression of joint damage, because damage can sometimes occur in as few as six months of the disease's onset. The challenge, though, is early diagnosis, because RA can be difficult to identify in its initial stages.

Soreness, stiffness and aching usually begin in the small joints of the feet, wrists and hands. It is especially common in the knuckles and middle joints of the hands. Pain and inflammation typically occur in the same joints on opposite sides of the body. Morning stiffness usually lasts for 45 minutes or longer, although the stiffness improves throughout the day. Fatigue is common.

RA may affect joints other than the hands, including the feet, knees, elbows, neck, shoulders, hips and ankles. Sometimes it affects organ systems such as the lungs or kidneys. Over time, if left untreated, the inflamed joints may become irreversibly damaged and deformed, although this is not always the case.

A doctor can determine if you have RA based on your symptoms, a physical examination, and results of x-rays and blood tests.

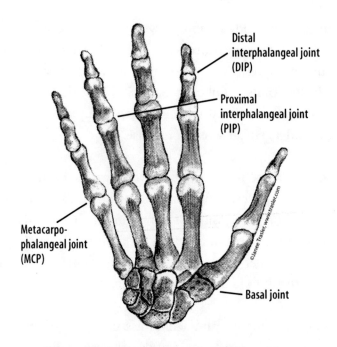

Distal
interphalangeal joint
(DIP)

Proximal
interphalangeal joint
(PIP)

Metacarpo-
phalangeal joint
(MCP)

Basal joint

Rheumatoid arthritis usually affects the small joints of the
hand, especially the MCPs,PIPs and wrist. Osteoarthritis
usually affects the DIPs, PIPs and basal joint.

Laboratory tests[3] can be very helpful in diagnosing RA.
One of the more common diagnostic blood tests for RA
screens for a substance in the blood called the rheumatoid factor (RF). Seventy-five percent of patients with RA have this
abnormal protein in their blood, although people who do not
have RA sometimes have RF in their blood. Some people with
the rheumatoid factor develop lumps under the skin called
rheumatoid nodules. The back of the elbow is a common
location. These nodules are usually not painful and typically
do not affect joint function.

---

3   Refer to Appendix B for additional information about common laboratory
    tests used in diagnosing and treating arthritis.

A newer screening test for RA, called the anti-cyclic citrullinated peptide (CCP) antibody test, was introduced in 2003. This test is considered to be more accurate than screening for the rheumatoid factor in patients where RA is suspected. The anti-CCP test screens for the presence of antibodies to CCP (also known as "CCP autoantibodies"). The test has been found to be effective in identifying patients with early, mild arthritis who may be at increased risk for developing a more severe, erosive form of RA.

IS IT OA OR RA?

Osteoarthritis (OA) and rheumatoid arthritis (RA) are the most common types of arthritis, but they involve different disease processes. OA is generally described as wear and tear on the joints. RA is a disease associated with an inflammatory process that can cause joint destruction and severe disability. With RA, early diagnosis and aggressive treatment can mean the difference between manageable discomfort and permanent disability.

	OA	RA
Joints involved	• Knees and hips • Hands and feet • Neck and lower back	Often begins in small joints: • Hands and wrists • Feet and knees May affect larger joints over time
Pattern of joint involvement	Random; one side of the body may predominate	May initially affect joints on just one side of the body, but usually affects the same joints on opposite sides of the body
If hand joints are involved	Affects distal finger joints (PIPs/DIPs) and basal joint*	Affects mid- and proximal finger joints (MCPs/PIPs)* and wrist
Morning stiffness	Brief: up to 30 minutes; pain worsens throughout the day with use	Prolonged: 45 minutes or longer; pain improves throughout the day

* See illustration on page 10.

Two additional laboratory tests are also usually ordered when RA is suspected. The first is the erythrocyte sedimentation rate (ESR) test. The second is the C-reactive protein (CRP) test. Elevated CRP and sedimentation rate are measures of joint inflammation, a key sign of RA.

Like osteoarthritis, there is no cure for rheumatoid arthritis. Treatment focuses on reducing inflammation and preventing further damage, which can help to relieve pain, improve joint mobility and decrease fatigue. Medications are prescribed to help in these areas and slow the progression of the disease. Diet, exercise and rest also play a role in improving range of motion, energy and sense of well-being.

JUVENILE CHRONIC ARTHRITIS: GROWING OLD TOO SOON

Arthritis can occur in children, and more than 150,000 American youngsters suffer with the disease. The disease has several common names — juvenile arthritis, juvenile rheumatoid arthritis, juvenile idiopathic arthritis and juvenile chronic arthritis (JCA). Regardless of what it is called, this form of the disease is always defined as arthritis in one or more joints before the age of 16.

Symptoms of juvenile chronic arthritis mimic those seen in adults: pain, stiffness, and swelling in affected joints. Juvenile chronic arthritis may also be accompanied by joint contracture (deformity), joint damage and changes in growth. Children may also show signs of weakness in their muscles, and tenderness in other soft tissues. However, the symptoms may also be elusive, changing from joint to joint and from day to day.

The key sign of juvenile chronic arthritis is symptoms of arthritis in one or more joints that last for six weeks or longer. The child may limp, be reluctant to use a limb, or lack the desire to play and be active. A definitive diagnosis of JCA is based primarily on symptoms, physical examination and laboratory studies.

Three Types of JCA

While joint inflammation is the common thread in all forms of juvenile chronic arthritis, three patterns of the disease are found among children diagnosed with the disease. Each of these three patterns has different possible outcomes. Therefore, each requires a different approach to treatment.

Pauciarticular onset JCA. Pauciarticular onset JCA affects four or fewer joints. It is the most common type of arthritis that affects children. More than half of children with JCA are afflicted with this form of the disease. It affects girls more frequently than boys. Younger children (ages 1 to 5) diagnosed with pauciarticular JCA are at increased risk for inflammatory eye disorders. Regular eye exams are recommended. The antinuclear antibody (ANA) is usually present in blood samples. Pauciarticular JCA in older children is more likely to affect multiple large joints such as the shoulders, hips and knees.

Systemic onset JCA. About 1 to 2 in 10 children with arthritis are diagnosed with systemic onset JCA. The illness begins with unexplained high fever spikes over 101°F (orally). The fever is often accompanied by a rash that comes and goes. Systemic onset JCA is often associated with an enlarged liver, spleen and lymph nodes, as well as growth retardation. Arthritis may not develop until several months into the illness. Long-term prognosis is based upon the severity of the arthritis.

Polyarticular JCA. Polyarticular JCA affects five or more joints, and often, many more. When laboratory tests are positive for the rheumatoid factor (RF), this pattern of the disease often mimics adult-type RA, with similar symptoms and the risk of progressive joint damage. Children with polyarticular JCA who test negative for RF are less likely to have significant joint involvement, and a better prognosis.

SPONDYLOARTHROPATHY

Spondyloarthropathy refers to a family of related diseases, including ankylosing spondylitis and psoriatic arthritis. These disorders are characterized by chronic inflammation, especially inflammation of the sacroiliac joints of the spine. Other joints and organs — particularly the eyes, skin and cardiovascular system — may also be involved.

The spondyloarthropathies share a common genetic marker known as HLA-B27, which can be detected in laboratory tests. Some forms of spondyloarthropathy also share a common pathology called enthesitis. Enthesitis is a chronic inflammation of the site where ligaments and tendons attach to bones.

The most common spondyloarthropathies are:

• Ankylosing spondylitis
• Psoriatic arthritis

- Reactive arthritis
- Inflammatory bowel disease associated with arthritis

Each of these is described in more detail below.

There is also a type of spondyloarthropathy called undifferentiated spondyloarthropathy. It has some but not all of the signs and symptoms of one of the specific spondyloarthropathies. Clinical investigators theorize that undifferentiated spondyloarthropathy may simply represent an early phase or incomplete form of ankylosing spondylitis or another spondyloarthropathy. However, clinical study data indicate that undifferentiated spondyloarthropathy may be a distinct form of spondyloarthropathy, just like ankylosing spondylitis, psoriatic arthritis or reactive arthritis.

ANKYLOSING SPONDYLITIS: A RARE ARTHRITIS OF THE SPINE

Ankylosing spondylitis is the most common spondyloarthropathy. The term "ankylosing spondylitis" means, literally, "inflamed spine that fuses together." It is a "seronegative" spondyloarthropathy, meaning that the rheumatoid factor (RF) is not present in the blood of patients with the disorder.

Ankylosing spondylitis affects primarily the spine and sacroiliac joints. The sacroiliac joints are the two joints located at the articulation of the sacrum and the ilium. The ilium is the largest bone of the pelvis.

People with ankylosing spondylitis often complain of prolonged morning stiffness in the low back and neck.

Ankylosing spondylitis can also cause inflammation of the tendons, eyes and lungs. Severe cases can lead to fusion of the spine and marked immobility.

Ankylosing spondylitis strikes mostly teen-aged males and young adult men. Women who are affected usually have a milder form of the disease. About 1 in 350,000 Americans has ankylosing spondylitis.

Early diagnosis is important to avoid joint damage, deformity and disability. But diagnosis is often delayed because the symptoms of ankylosing spondylitis mirror that of common back problems. Laboratory tests can aid an accurate diagnosis. Markers for the disease include an elevated sedimentation rate

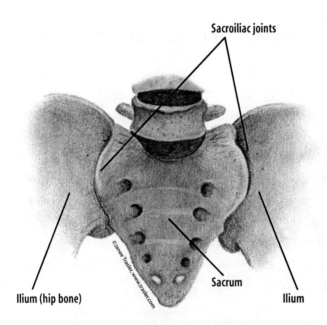

Ankylosing spondylitis affects both the spine and the sacroiliac joints.

and elevated C-reactive protein, both of which indicate inflammation, as well as a positive HLA-B27 test. Arthritic changes may also be seen on x-rays and in bone scans.

Treatment for ankylosing spondylitis consists of anti-inflammatory medications or TNF blockers, aerobic exercise and physical therapy. Rehabilitation focuses on proper posture, exercises to strengthen the back and abdomen, breathing exercises to enhance lung capacity, and other exercises to maintain range of motion. Ongoing physical therapy is critical to avoiding a stiff or "ankylosed" spine, which can severely limit mobility and cause permanent disability.

PSORIATIC ARTHRITIS: ARTHRITIS INVOLVING THE JOINTS AND SKIN

Psoriatic arthritis is an inflammatory condition that is related to the skin condition psoriasis. It is often accompanied by tell-tale skin patches of raised red areas that have a crusty, silvery scale. The skin lesions usually appear on the scalp, elbows, knees or lower back, but they may appear anywhere on the body.

About 10 percent of Americans with psoriasis also have the arthritic form of the disease. Abnormalities of the fingernails and toenails in patients with psoriasis increase the likelihood that they will develop the arthritic form of the disease. Psoriatic arthritis strikes men and women equally, and is usually diagnosed between the ages of 30 and 50. Among people who have first-degree relatives (parents and siblings) with psoriatic arthritis, there is an increased risk of developing the disease.

Psoriatic arthritis is a seronegative spondyloarthropathy. It is diagnosed through physical examination, x-rays and laboratory tests. Lab test abnormalities seen with psoriatic arthritis often mimic RA, except the rheumatoid factor is usually absent and HLA-B27 is present. Psoriatic changes in the skin and nails must also be present before a definitive diagnosis of psoriatic arthritis is made.

Treatment focuses on medications to relieve the inflammation, including NSAIDs, Azulfidine® (sulfasalazine), methotrexate and TNF blockers.

Five Patterns of Psoriatic Arthritis

There are five types of psoriatic arthritis. Each is distinguished by the pattern of the involved joints, but all are associated with skin psoriasis.

Symmetric psoriatic arthritis. Symmetric psoriatic arthritis is the most common form of psoriatic arthritis. It involves pain and swelling in many joints, particularly the small joints of the fingers and toes. It is similar to rheumatoid arthritis in that it affects the same joints on opposite sides of the body.

Asymmetric psoriatic arthritis. Asymmetric psoriatic arthritis involves a few joints of the extremities, but in a random pattern, such as the fingers on the left hand and toes on the right foot.

Psoriatic spondylitis. Psoriatic spondylitis affects specific joints of the lower spine called the sacroiliac joints.

Distal interphalangeal predominant psoriatic arthritis. This form of psoriatic arthritis primarily involves the joints closest to the nails of the fingers and toes. It may also affect other joints. This form of the disease often involves changes in the nails, including pitting, splitting or degeneration.

Arthritis mutilans. The fifth type of psoriatic arthritis is arthritis mutilans. It is a very rare, painful and destructive form of psoriatic arthritis that involves inflammation where tendons and ligaments attach to the bone (a condition called enthesitis).

REACTIVE ARTHRITIS

Reactive arthritis is a type of arthritis that occurs in response to an environmental "trigger," such as an infection, trauma or injury (thus the term "reactive"). Like ankylosing spondylitis and psoriatic arthritis, reactive arthritis is a "seronegative" spondyloarthropathy. This means that the rheumatoid factor (RF) is not present in the blood of patients with the disorder.

Reactive arthritis was formerly called Reiter's syndrome. The condition is characterized by inflammation that typically affects three areas: (1) the joints, especially the sacroiliac joints of the spine; (2) the urethra, the tube that drains urine from the body; and (3) the eyelids and membranes that cover the eye. (This condition is called conjunctivitis.) A skin rash and inflammation of the mucous membranes, such as the mouth, may also present.

Symptoms of reactive arthritis usually last for several months to a year. However, symptoms can come and go. In a small number of reactive arthritis patients, the symptoms develop into a chronic form of the disease.

A doctor can determine if you have reactive arthritis based on your symptoms, medical history, physical examination and blood tests. Blood tests may be used to rule out other types of arthritis as well as to determine if a bacterial infection is present. The genetic marker HLA B-27 is found in the blood of a majority of people with this disorder.

X-rays may be ordered to assess the presence of inflammation in the sacroiliac joints of the spine, but x-rays are usually inconclusive in patients in the early stages of reactive arthritis.

Treatment for reactive arthritis includes NSAIDs to relieve inflammation, as well as rest and joint protection. Your physician may also recommend physical therapy or exercise program to improve mobility of affected joints.

INFLAMMATORY BOWEL DISEASE ASSOCIATED WITH ARTHRITIS

Inflammatory bowel disease (IBD) has two forms: Crohn's disease and ulcerative colitis. Both disorders are thought to be associated with an overactive immune system, which causes inflammation of some portion of the gastrointestinal tract. About 25 percent of people diagnosed with IBD also develop arthritis. A small number of patients also develop inflammation of other parts of the body, such as the skin, eyes or liver. Men and women are affected equally by IBD-associated arthritis, usually between the ages of 25 and 45.

Ulcerative colitis and Crohn's disease have similar signs and symptoms. Diagnosis is aided by physical examination, as well as results of blood tests that confirm the presence of HLA-B27. Treatment for the bowel symptoms depends upon whether the patient has Crohn's disease or ulcerative colitis. Treatment of the underlying bowel disease often helps the arthritis. Other common treatments for the arthritis include injecting the joints with corticosteroids, oral corticosteroids, Azulfidine® (sulfasalazine) and tumor necrosis factor (TNF) blockers.

Crohn's Disease

Crohn's disease may cause inflammation of any part of the gastrointestinal tract from the mouth to the rectum, although it usually involves the large intestine (colon) or a portion of the small intestine called the ileum. The inflammation involves all layers of the intestinal wall, which may cause scarring and narrowing of the bowel. Patients with Crohn's disease often complain of symptoms that are similar to ulcerative colitis: fever, weight loss and loss of appetite. Joint inflammation — particularly of the knees, ankles and wrists — may also occur, especially at the same time that the bowel symptoms flare. Some patients with Crohn's disease also develop ankylosing spondylitis, which causes back pain.

Crohn's disease is often treated with 5-amino salicylic acid products, such as Azulfidine® (sulfasalazine), which helps to control both the bowel symptoms and the arthritis. Corticosteroids and immunosuppressive drugs such as Imuran® (azathioprine), as well as the TNF blocker Remicade®, are alternative drug therapies that can be effective in treating Crohn's disease. In severe cases, surgery may be required to remove the diseased portion of the bowel. While this can eliminate the bothersome bowel symptoms, it may not help with the arthritis, particularly arthritis that affects the spine.

Ulcerative Colitis

Ulcerative colitis causes inflammation and erosion of the lining of the colon. The disease usually begins at the rectum and moves up into the large intestine. Patients with ulcerative colitis often complain of symptoms similar to Crohn's disease — abdominal cramping, fever and weight loss. Rectal bleeding may also occur. When arthritis is involved, one or more joints may be affected, and the symptoms often move from joint to joint. The most commonly affected joints include the knees and ankles, but any joint may be involved. Unlike RA, involved joints are not typically damaged by the disease process.

As with Crohn's disease, ulcerative colitis is treated with Azulfidine® (sulfasalazine), corticosteroids or immunosuppressive drugs. Surgery can be an effective treatment in severe cases, and unlike Crohn's disease, removal of the diseased portion of the bowel usually eliminates the arthritis.

GOUT: A COMMON AND TREATABLE FORM OF ARTHRITIS

Gout affects more than 2 million Americans. It is caused by deposits of uric acid — a white, odorless crystal that accumulates in the body and causes redness and swelling of the joints. Attacks come on suddenly and are painful. The big toe, ankle and knee are common sites of involvement. While gout can occur in men and women of all ages, it rarely occurs in women before menopause.

To obtain a definite diagnosis of gout, fluid must be removed from an affected joint and tested for the presence of uric acid. The reason for a joint fluid test rather than a blood test is two-fold. First, the uric acid level in the blood may be normal even when gout is present. Second, a high level of uric acid in the blood by itself does not necessarily signify the presence of gout.

Medications and diet are often culprits of gout attacks. Certain substances in medications and food can increase levels of uric acid in the blood. Diuretics such as Lasix® and hydrochlorothiazide, which are used to treat high blood pressure and edema (fluid retention), can increase the risk of gout attacks. Aspirin also increases uric acid levels and can worsen attacks.

Foods with high purine levels also increase uric acid levels in the blood. So changing your diet may help to prevent attacks. Avoiding sweetbreads, herring, mussels and sardines can be helpful. So, too, can avoiding alcoholic beverages, especially beer, heavy wines and champagne. Results of a study published in the *New England Journal of Medicine* indicate that a diet that includes dairy products and vegetables may help to prevent gout.[4] Obesity and overeating or "bingeing" have been associated with gout, so maintaining a reasonable weight may also be a preventative measure.

---

4   Choi HK, Atkinson K, Karlson EW. Purine-rich foods, dairy and protein intake, and the risk of gout in men. *N Engl J Med.* 2004;350:1093-1103.

If frequent gout attacks persist despite changes in medications or diet, your doctor may prescribe certain drugs to prevent flare-ups. These include colchicine, Benemid® (probenecid) or Zyloprim® (allopurinol).

LUPUS ERYTHEMATOSUS: "MARK OF THE WOLF"

Lupus erythematosus (pronounced loo-pus air-re-them-a-toe-sus) is an autoimmune disorder like RA. The disease was named by clinicians who observed that the skin problems that often signal the condition resembled the facial markings of a wolf (lupus means wolf; erythematosus means redness).

The cause of lupus is generally unknown. Researchers theorize that the most likely culprit is a genetic disposition toward the disease, combined with a subsequent exposure to some environmental insult or infection that leads to a "confused" immune system that attacks the body's own tissues. Up to 5 percent of sisters and daughters of patients with lupus may also develop the disease. It is not uncommon for relatives of lupus patients to have abnormal antibodies in their blood, but with no symptoms of the disease. Lower levels of anti-nuclear antibodies (ANA) are often found when RA is also present.

It used to be that only the most severe cases of lupus were diagnosed. Now, due to the sensitivity of newer ANA blood tests, milder cases of lupus are diagnosed more quickly. Most people with lupus live a normal life with few changes in lifestyle. Nevertheless, detecting the condition early allows patients to be monitored for evidence of more serious illness, and treated appropriately.

Treatment of lupus is based on the underlying symptoms. Plaquenil® (hydroxychloroquine sulfate), which is also used in RA, may help to control the skin and joint symptoms of lupus, as well as the fatigue. When internal organs such as the kidneys, heart or lungs are involved, stronger medications may be prescribed. These include Imuran® (azathioprine), CellCept® (mycophenolate mofetil) or Cytoxan® (cyclophosphamide). These medications may be very effective, but they can pose an increased risk of potential side effects.

Some people with lupus do not have to take medications regularly. Prescription drugs (such as corticosteroids) may be ordered as needed for flare-up of symptoms.

Four Types of Lupus

There are four types of lupus. All feature the tell-tale skin rash that is the hallmark of the disorder. None of the four types of lupus are infectious. Nor are they a type of cancer or malignancy. Like RA, people with lupus have an overactive immune system. The number of cases of lupus in the United States is unknown, but experts estimate that up to 1.5 million people may be affected with the disease. Ninety percent of lupus patients are women.

Drug-induced lupus. Drug-induced lupus is a rare condition caused from long-term exposure to certain medications. The condition clears up once the offending medication is stopped. However, the presence of anti-nuclear antibodies (ANA), a marker for lupus, may continue to show in blood tests for a year or more.

Discoid lupus. Discoid lupus is identified by a skin rash with raised, red, scaling areas. These lesions sometimes leave scars, and are typically seen on the face, scalp and other sun-exposed areas. Most people with discoid lupus do not have internal organ involvement, as is seen with the systemic form of the disease.

Subacute lupus. Like discoid lupus, subacute lupus is also associated with a skin rash with raised, red scaly patches. However, unlike discoid lupus, this form of the disease does not scar.

Systemic lupus erythematosus (SLE). In the 1890s, the famed physician Sir William Osler observed that internal organs — or systems — can also be involved in addition to skin changes associated with lupus. Thus, the term systemic lupus erythematosus (SLE) was coined.

Symptoms of SLE include arthritis, rash, and flu-like symptoms such as aching joints and muscles and fatigue. Infection and sunlight may trigger lupus, but symptoms seem to come and go for no apparent reason. This makes the condition harder to diagnose.

SLE commonly affects the heart or lungs, where there is usually an inflammation of the organ's lining. This may cause chest pain, especially with breathing. The kidneys may also be involved in SLE. Patients may have no symptoms, but a urine test can detect evidence of inflammation. Other systems and regions affected by SLE may include the bone marrow (blood cells), the brain and blood vessels.

Lupus Isn't Always a Clear-Cut Diagnosis

Lupus can be difficult to diagnose. The American College of Rheumatology established 11 criteria to help identify the disorder. A person with lupus usually has four or more of the following symptoms:

1.	Malar "butterfly" rash on the cheeks.
2.	Discoid skin lesions.
3.	Sun sensitivity, where a rash develops from exposure to sun or UV light.
4.	Mouth sores, usually on the roof or back of the mouth (typically not painful).
5.	Arthritis, with prolonged morning stiffness, usually up to an hour, improving as the day goes on.
6.	Abnormal urine test showing large amounts of protein.
7.	A history of seizures or psychiatric problems.
8.	Sharp pain during breathing due to inflammation of the lining of the lungs or heart, which worsens with deep inhalations (pleurisy).
9.	Low white blood count, low platelet count or evidence of anemia.
10.	The presence of antibodies to double-strand DNA (ds-DNA), or of Smith (Sm) antibodies which are specific for diagnosing lupus.
11.	A positive anti-nuclear antibody (ANA) test. 98 percent of people with lupus have this antibody.

SJÖGREN'S SYNDROME: PAINFULLY DRY EYES AND MOUTH

Sjögren's (pronounced show-grens) syndrome is an autoimmune condition. The body's immune system turns against itself, subsequently destroying the exocrine glands that produce tears, saliva and mucus.

The condition was first described in 1933 by the Swedish physician Henrik Sjögren. He reported women whose arthritis was associated with dryness of their eyes and mouth.

When these symptoms occur without any other rheumatologic condition, it is described as "primary" Sjögren's syndrome. When it occurs with another rheumatologic condition such as lupus, RA or scleroderma, it is called "secondary" Sjögren's syndrome.

The cause of Sjögren's syndrome is unknown, although scientists believe that genetically predisposed patients may come in contact with a virus or certain bacteria that triggers the immune response. This response inactivates tear and saliva glands. The result is uncomfortably dry eyes and dry mouth.

People with Sjögren's often describe eye irritation and grittiness, as if there is sand in their eye. A burning sensation in the mouth or throat is also common, as is a hoarse voice or difficulty swallowing because food sticks to the dry tissue. Enlarged or infected glands that cause pain are also common, as is vaginal dryness among women. Many patients also complain of aching and fatigue.

Sjögren's syndrome affects approximately 1 in 2500 people, but the condition is frequently overlooked.

A blood test can help to diagnosis the condition. Most people with Sjögren's syndrome have at least one antibody in their blood that is a specific marker for the disease. The markers that may be present in Sjögren's syndrome include:

- Antibodies to the rheumatoid factor (RF), which are found in RA and Sjögren's syndrome

- Those to the anti-nuclear antibodies (ANA), which are found in RA, Sjögren's syndrome, lupus and scleroderma
- Those to anti-Sjögren's syndrome A (anti-SSA or "Ro"), which are found in RA, Sjögren's syndrome and lupus
- Those to anti-Sjögren's syndrome B (anti-SSB or "La"), which is diagnostic for primary Sjögren's syndrome

Definitive diagnosis is based on a thorough history and physical examination as well as the results of the laboratory tests to detect the presence of the antibodies that are characteristic of Sjögren's syndrome. A biopsy of the minor salivary gland found in the lips may also be performed.

There is no treatment that is capable of producing normal glandular conditions, so treatment focuses on treating symptoms of dry eyes and mouth. Lubricants, as well as medications that decrease inflammation, stimulate moisture and help patients to feel better.

SCLERODERMA: AN AUTOIMMUNE DISORDER THAT AFFECTS THE SKIN

Scleroderma is not well understood, but is believed to be an autoimmune condition. The term "scleroderma" means, literally, "hard skin," which refers to the smooth, tightened or thickened areas of skin that are a common sign of the disorder.

Scleroderma is a relatively rare disease. It is estimated that approximately 300,000 Americans have been diagnosed with the disorder. The disease affects all age groups, but is most commonly seen in women between the ages of 25 and 55.

Diagnosing scleroderma can be difficult because the symptoms mimic many other diseases. A definite diagnosis is based on a medical history, physical examination and blood tests. Almost all patients with scleroderma have anti-nuclear antibodies in their blood. In addition, a number of scleroderma-specific antibodies may be present in the blood, which can facilitate diagnosis. A skin biopsy can be helpful in diagnosing scleroderma, but is not able to differentiate whether the limited or diffuse form of the disease is involved.

There is no cure for scleroderma. Treatment is based on relieving symptoms, particularly those of dry skin and joint inflammation and pain. There are two forms of scleroderma: localized and systemic.

Localized Scleroderma

Localized scleroderma typically affects only a few areas of the skin or several muscles and joints. It is more common in children than adults, and rarely develops into the systemic form of the disease. Localized scleroderma is also known as morphea.

Systemic Scleroderma

The second form of scleroderma is called systemic scleroderma. It is also known as systemic sclerosis. This form of the disease involves the skin, as well as the underlying connective tissues, including blood vessels, muscles, bones and joints. Systemic scleroderma may also affect major organs, such as the heart, lungs and kidneys.

A diagnosis of systemic scleroderma is usually further classified as one of three types:

Limited scleroderma. This type of systemic scleroderma typically develops slowly over a period of years. It usually affects the skin only on the hands and face. People with limited scleroderma may experience Raynaud's phenomenon (explained below) for years before the thickened, hard skin symptoms characteristic of scleroderma develop.

Limited scleroderma is sometimes called CREST syndrome. The term CREST is an acronym for the five major characteristics of the disorder:

- C – Calcinosis. This refers to the formation of calcium deposits under the skin. These are seen as hard, white areas on the skin, usually on the elbows, knees or fingers. Not all patients with limited scleroderma have calcinosis.

- R – Raynaud's phenomenon. Raynaud's phenomenon is a condition in which the small blood vessels of the fingers or toes narrow in response to cold temperatures or emotional upset. As the vessels contract, the skin turns white, then blue. As blood flow returns, the skin become reddened. Raynaud's (pronounced ray-noze) phenomenon can occasionally damage the tissue, which may result in skin ulcers, scarring or gangrene.

- E – Esophageal involvement. This is most often described as difficulty in swallowing, due to a poorly functioning muscle in the lower part of the esophagus. This condition can lead to stomach acid backflow into

the esophagus, which can cause heartburn, inflammation and scarring.

- S – Sclerodactyly. This refers to the thickening and tightening of the skin of the fingers, which results in a shiny
and slightly puffy appearance. Skin tightening can limit
mobility.

- T – Telangietasia. This refers to small areas of redness that
most frequently appear on the face, hands and mouth.

Diffuse scleroderma. Diffuse scleroderma typically develops over a shorter time frame than the limited type of the
disease. The skin symptoms occur quickly and spread over
most of the body. Skin thickening may affect the face, chest and
stomach, as well as the upper arms and legs. Like RA, the
affected areas are often symmetric. This means that if one side
of the body or a limb is involved, the other side is also affected.
Diffuse scleroderma may also affect the heart, lungs or kidneys.

Diffuse scleroderma is often cyclical. The disease may be
active for several years, followed by a quiet period during
which skin symptoms remain stable and joint pain and
fatigue lessen.

Sine scleroderma. In recent years, a third type of systemic
scleroderma has been identified to describe the form of the
disease that causes changes to the internal organs, but without
hardening or tightening of the skin. This type of systemic sclerosis is called "sine scleroderma." In Latin, "sine" means
"without," which refers to the lack of skin involvement in this
form of systemic scleroderma.

FIBROMYALGIA: "I HURT ALL OVER"

Fibromyalgia (pronounced fi-bro-my-al-juh) is a very common and often undiagnosed cause of musculoskeletal pain. The condition affects nearly 4 million americans, mostly women between the ages of 20 and 50, but it can occur in people of all ages.

People with fibromyalgia typically complain of hurting all over and non-restful sleep. Even with adequate amounts of sleep, people with fibromyalgia still wake up feeling unrested. The lack of restful sleep seems to exacerbate or worsen the symptoms, resulting in a vicious cycle of increasing fatigue and pain.

There is no laboratory test to diagnose fibromyalgia. It is often a "diagnosis of exclusion," meaning that your doctor will try to rule out other causes of the symptoms. Conditions that must first be ruled out include lupus, rheumatoid arthritis, thyroid disease, and sleep apnea. A diagnosis of fibromyalgia may be confirmed by identifying a number of "tender points," which are certain areas of the body that are painful to the touch.

There is no cure for fibromyalgia, but it is not a deforming or life-threatening disease. The most important aspect of treatment is education. Learning about the condition and what causes the symptoms is very important in recovery. Aerobic exercise for 20 to 30 minutes three or four times a week can also be useful for improving sleep quality.

Many people with rheumatoid arthritis, lupus and other arthritic conditions may also have fibromyalgia. In fact, fibromyalgia should be considered a possible explanation for symptoms in arthritis patients whose pain is not improving despite improvement in joint swelling.

CHAPTER 3

Understanding Arthritis Therapy

There is no cure for any of the 100 non-infectious types of arthritis. Therapy is aimed at treating pain and swelling, and relieving other symptoms as they arise.

In rheumatoid arthritis (RA) in particular, the goal of treatment is to reduce joint inflammation in an effort to slow progression of the disease and prevent damage, deformity and disability. A comprehensive treatment plan that includes medications, physical rehabilitation, adequate rest and good nutrition can help you maintain a lifestyle that is as pain-free as possible.

For decades, the only real advance in treating RA was to treat it sooner and more aggressively in hopes of preventing joint damage. The status quo in RA treatment changed for the better in 1988 when the U.S. Food and Drug Administration (FDA) approved a drug called methotrexate for RA; and dramatically so in the late 1990s and into the new millennium, when nine new medicines for arthritis were introduced, five of them specifically for RA.

But before we talk about this revolution in RA therapy, it is important to understand how physicians approach RA treatment.

NSAIDS: THE FIRST-LINE TREATMENT FOR ARTHRITIS

Non-steroidal anti-inflammatory drugs, or NSAIDs, are the first line of treatment for most types of arthritis, including RA. NSAIDs block the effects of two enzymes called cyclooxygenase-1 and cyclooxygenase-2, or COX-1 and COX-2.

COX-1 protects the stomach lining and maintains platelet function, which controls normal blood clotting. COX-2 is involved with joint inflammation and helps to maintain blood flow to the kidneys. Blocking COX-1 and COX-2 helps to decrease the pain and swelling of arthritis, but may also cause adverse effects, including stomach ulcers, bleeding and kidney damage.

NSAIDs usually provide some pain relief within the first day or two of treatment, but it may take over a month to get full benefit from these drugs. Commonly prescribed NSAIDs include Motrin® or Advil® (ibuprofen), Voltaren® (diclofenac), Lodine® (etodolac), Relafen® (nabumetone), and Aleve® or Naprosyn® (naproxen).

NSAIDs can be effective in relieving symptoms of arthritis but they do not slow the progression of RA. Nor do they prevent joint deformity. People who are 60 years or older are particularly at risk for potentially severe gastrointestinal problems with NSAIDs, including stomach ulcers or gastrointestinal bleeding. Often, older people taking NSAIDs have no symptoms prior to developing bleeding, which can be severe or life-threatening. Liver abnormalities are also not uncommon in people taking NSAIDs, but the abnormalities often correct themselves when the NSAID is discontinued. On occasion, however, permanent liver damage may occur.

Many NSAIDs can be purchased over-the-counter. Stronger dosages of NSAIDs for severe pain and inflammation are available by prescription.

DMARDS: THE MAINSTAY OF RA THERAPY

In addition to NSAIDs, physicians also rely on a second category of drugs to treat RA. These drugs are called disease-modifying anti-rheumatic drugs, or DMARDs. DMARDs can help to slow the course of RA, and sometimes prevent damage to joints.

Research has shown that the role of DMARDs in RA is an important one. In a study[5] conducted in the 1990s, researchers began using a tool called the Health Assessment Questionnaire (HAQ) to evaluate patient outcomes in RA.

What was learned with regard to RA was alarming. Nearly half of RA patients stopped working within five to 10 years of the disease's onset due to disability. Researchers also noted that joint erosions occur early in the disease, usually within the first 24 months, and that RA can shorten life expectancies.

---

5   Pincus T, Brooks RH, Callahan LF. Prediction of long-term mortality in patients with rheumatoid arthritis according to simple questionnaire and joint count measures. *Ann Intern Med.* 1994;120(1):26-34.

All of these factors contributed to a new philosophy within the medical and scientific communities about how best to treat RA. The methodical approach of trying a variety of NSAIDs before moving on to DMARDs was replaced by early, aggressive treatment with DMARDs to prevent or postpone the joint deformity and disability.

Today, physicians usually begin DMARD therapy very soon after RA is diagnosed. Unlike quick-acting NSAIDs, it may take up to six months to see benefit with some DMARDs. To further relieve pain and inflammation before the DMARDs begin to work, NSAIDs or low-dose corticosteroids may be prescribed in addition to DMARDs. This is known as "bridge therapy."

DMARD therapy may begin with a single drug or a combination of drugs. How DMARDs work is not well understood, but it is thought that DMARDs control inflammation by acting on some component of the immune system. An overactive immune system is implicated in RA, and drugs like DMARDs that help to regulate, or "modulate," the immune system can help to decrease joint swelling and pain, and prevent damage and deformity. However, some of these medications require close attention and follow-up by a physician to avoid suppressing the immune system to the degree that it is unable to fight off infection. Such a scenario can put a patient at risk for a serious or opportunistic infection.

DMARDs can also have adverse side effects. These range from a mild rash or mouth sores to more serious conditions like blood toxicities or damage to the lungs, kidneys, or gastrointestinal system, including the liver. People taking DMARDs should be checked periodically by their doctor.

Regularly scheduled blood tests and physical exams are important in monitoring overall health while taking DMARDs.

The Key DMARDs for RA

A number of DMARDs are commonly used in RA therapy. Five of these drugs have received FDA approval specifically for rheumatoid arthritis:

- Methotrexate (sold as Rheumatrex®). Methotrexate, which is also abbreviated as MTX, is the most widely used DMARD for RA and psoriatic arthritis
- Plaquenil® (hydroxychloroquine sulfate)
- Azulfidine® (sulfasalazine)
- Injectable gold or gold sodium thiomalate (sold as Myochrysine®)
- Imuran® (azathioprine)

A sixth drug, Minocin® (minocycline hydrochloride)[6], is also used sometimes as a DMARD to treat RA, although it has not been FDA-approved for this disease.

METHOTREXATE: THE GOLD STANDARD OF ARTHRITIS THERAPY

Methotrexate (MTX) was approved by the FDA in 1988 for the treatment of rheumatoid arthritis in adults. Rheumatologists and other physicians borrowed this treatment from oncologists who had been using MTX in much

---

6 Although the FDA has not approved Minocin® (minocycline hydrochloride) for use in RA, some physicians may prescribe it for this or other conditions. The practice of prescribing prescription drugs for unapproved uses is called "off label" use. Off-label prescribing is a common practice.

higher doses since the 1950s to treat cancer, primarily child-hood leukemia and other lymphomas.

The use of low-dose methotrexate to treat RA and associ-ated conditions was considered to be the biggest breakthrough in the treatment of arthritis since the 1930s, when corticos-teroid therapy was introduced. Today, methotrexate is considered the gold standard of arthritis treatment, particularly in RA. Its demonstrated safety and effectiveness is the standard against which all new therapies for arthritis are measured.

Uses of Methotrexate

Methotrexate can be very effective in treating RA, psoriatic arthritis, and more recently, lupus. It is also effective in treat-ing juvenile chronic arthritis. Numerous clinical studies have shown that joint pain and inflammation improve greatly with the drug. This is generally the case even for patients who had not had success with anti-inflammatories such as ibuprofen, aspirin, naproxen, as well as other RA-specific DMARDs.

Benefits of Methotrexate

Methotrexate is a very effective anti-inflammatory drug in low doses, without much of the toxicity or side effects of the high doses used in chemotherapy. In arthritis treatment, sig-nificant relief with low-dose MTX occurs relatively quickly — within eight to 12 weeks of starting the drug. Maximum ben-efit is usually attained by six months.

Methotrexate is a convenient therapy. It is taken once a week as a single, easy-to-swallow pill that offers long-lasting relief. Patients who occasionally skip a week of methotrexate because they forget or are traveling typically do so without harm or loss of relief.

Methotrexate has demonstrated such effectiveness in arthritis therapy that it is the anchor drug for nearly all successful combination drug regimens. Studies have also shown that some patients are better able to continue taking methotrexate over the long term than other DMARDs. Methotrexate also has a lower probability of being discontinued due to lack of effectiveness than other DMARDs, and discontinuation due to toxicity issues was less frequent and occurred later in the course of treatment than any other DMARD except Plaquenil® (hydroxychloroquine sulfate). Clinical data also indicate that RA patients taking methotrexate have better survival rates and a lower incidence of death due to cardiovascular events.

Methotrexate is also cost effective. The pill form costs about $160 per month, and is covered by most insurance prescription drug plans. Methotrexate is also available in an injectable form, which is about one-fifth of the cost of the pills.

MTX Dosage and Regimen

Methotrexate is taken as a single dose once a week. The once-weekly dosage should not be exceeded, even if you forget and miss a dose.

The standard initial dose for rheumatoid arthritis and related conditions is usually 7.5 mg to 10 mg weekly. This weekly dosage may be increased to a maximum dosage of 20 mg given orally, or 25 mg given by injection.

Contraindications to Methotrexate

Methotrexate should not be prescribed to people who have a known sensitivity to the drug. Nor should it be taken by women who are pregnant, nursing, or not using an effective method of birth control. Methotrexate is also not suitable for people with RA or psoriatic arthritis who also have a blood disorder, kidney disease, liver disease, alcoholism or an immune-system deficiency.

Side Effects of Methotrexate

The most common side effects of methotrexate are nausea, lack of appetite, vomiting, diarrhea and painful mouth ulcers. Other side effects include headache, dizziness, mood swings, memory impairment, fatigue, post-therapy flares, fever, impotence, rash, weight loss and sun sensitivity.

Physicians have several alternatives to help decrease unwanted side effects. These include decreasing the dose, dividing the dose over a 24-hour period, and administering the drug by injection rather than by mouth. Methotrexate is a folic acid antagonist that works by interfering with folic acid function. (Folic acid is a vitamin involved in cell growth.) Your physician should recommend at least 1 mg folic acid supplement daily to help prevent certain serious side effects without decreasing the effectiveness of the drug. Folinic acid, which is also known as leucovorin, can be even more helpful in minimizing side effects when taken eight to 12 hours after methotrexate therapy.

Potential Drug Interactions

There are a number of other drugs that may increase the toxic effects of methotrexate. These include but are not limited to sulfa-based antibiotics such as Bactrim® and Septra® (trimethoprim sulfamethoxazole). These drugs should be avoided while taking methotrexate because they may increase methotrexate's toxic effect on the bone marrow, where new blood cells are made.

MTX and Infection

Methotrexate is a powerful drug, but if used wisely and with monitoring, it can also be a safe and effective therapy. Taking methotrexate during an infection may increase the risk of bone marrow depression, causing the white blood cell count to drop. This can lead to serious infections.

There are a number of things that the patient and physician can do to minimize the risk of bone marrow depression and more serious problems. These include:

- Daily supplementation with folic acid
- Careful monitoring of blood cell counts and blood chemistry every four to eight weeks
- Dose adjustments for patients with kidney disease or low white blood cell counts
- Avoiding sulfa-based drugs, as noted above

Patients should always discontinue methotrexate and notify their physician if symptoms of infection develop while taking methotrexate. If you are scheduled for surgery, your doctor may recommend that methotrexate should also be discontinued prior to and for a short time following surgery due to the possible increased risk of infection.

MTX and Lung/Liver Toxicity

Methotrexate may also cause lung or liver toxicity in some patients. There is a small but definite chance of developing a life-threatening pulmonary reaction to methotrexate. For an unknown reason, inflammation may develop in the lungs, causing shortness of breath, fever and cough. If a patient develops these symptoms while taking methotrexate, the drug should be discontinued immediately and the physician notified.

Methotrexate is also associated with a small but increased risk of liver damage, such as cirrhosis. Minor elevation of liver function is common among patients taking methotrexate. But it can also indicate a problem, so regular monitoring is an important part of therapy. Cirrhosis and severe liver damage is rare in RA, but more common in psoriasis patients. It is recommended that psoriasis patients have a liver biopsy when they have taken a cumulative total of 1500 mg of methotrexate, and at every 1500 mg interval thereafter.

Screening for prior exposure to hepatitis (e.g., hepatitis B or C) or other liver disorders is recommended before starting on methotrexate. This can help to identify patients most at risk for developing liver disease. To further minimize the risk of liver disease while taking methotrexate, patients should avoid alcohol and take a daily folic acid supplement.

MTX and Pregnancy

Methotrexate has been shown to cause miscarriages and birth defects. It is strongly recommended that both the males and females use a reliable method of birth control while taking methotrexate and for at least 90 days after discontinuing the drug. (In fact, your physician may recommend that you use two forms of reliable birth control, such as birth control pills and condoms.) Because the effect of methotrexate on nursing infants is unknown, breastfeeding is not recommended while taking the drug.

You should not begin methotrexate therapy if you are pregnant, suspect you are pregnant, or are considering pregnancy. Contact your physician immediately if you become pregnant, your period is late, or you want to begin trying to conceive.

MTX and Fertility

There is currently no evidence that methotrexate affects fertility in men or women. Nor does available data suggest that methotrexate increases the risk of male-mediated fetal damage. However, to minimize the possible risk of fetal damage, men wanting to father a child should consider discontinuing methotrexate for at least three months before trying to conceive a child.

MTX and Cancer

There have been rare reports of patients who developed lymphoma while taking methotrexate. Many cases went into remission when methotrexate was discontinued. At this time, the true incidence of malignancy associated with methotrexate use is unclear, although scientific data have failed to show that methotrexate increases the incidence of cancer other than lymphoma.

COMBINATION DMARD THERAPY

In the past 20 years, rheumatologists have begun to use combinations of drugs to treat RA and psoriatic arthritis. Two or more DMARDs are sometimes used together in an attempt to bring about a more dramatic response. This drug regimen is called "combination therapy." Common combinations include methotrexate/cyclosporine, as well as methotrexate/ hydroxychloroquine/sulfasalazine (which is called "triple therapy" because three drugs are combined). More recently, the combination of methotrexate and doxycycline is being studied. The most successful combination therapy used today typically includes methotrexate or a TNF inhibitor (described in Chapter 5) as the anchor drug.

Like DMARDs used individually, combined DMARDs may also cause adverse side effects. Your physician will likely want to closely monitor your progress and your health status while on a combination drug regimen.

CORTICOSTEROIDS: A BRIDGE THERAPY FOR ARTHRITIS

A third type of drug sometimes used to treat RA is corticosteroids. This type of steroid is very different than steroids used to improve muscle strength. The anabolic type of steroids sometimes used inappropriately by athletes is similar to the male hormone testosterone. The corticosteroids used in arthritis treatment are naturally-occurring substances produced by the adrenal glands.

Corticosteroids were one of the first drugs used in RA therapy, dating back to the 1940s. They were hailed as "miracle drugs" at the time. In fact, the 1950 Nobel prize in medicine was awarded to Dr. Philip S. Henach, the physician at the Mayo Clinic in Rochester, Minnesota, who discovered the naturally-produced adrenal substance that came to be known as "cortisone." (Adrenaline is a steroid-like hormone made by the adrenal gland at times of extreme injury, stress or illness.)

Corticosteroids are a potent anti-inflammatory agent and can provide substantial relief to patients with arthritis and related conditions. Commonly prescribed oral corticosteroids for arthritis include Deltasone® and Orasone® (prednisone), Medrol® (methylprednisolone) and prednisolone.

Clinical studies have shown that low doses of prednisone, up to 7.5 mg a day, may be helpful in preventing some of the damage in the joints of people with RA. Ideally, if corticosteroids are prescribed, the lowest possible dose of corticosteroids should be given. Even so, these low doses are not without potential side effects, especially when taken over a period of time. Side effects of low doses include, but are not limited to, the possibility of damage to bones (osteoporosis) and eyes (cataract formation), as well as weight gain.

Due to the possibility of side effects, a low-dose corticosteroid may be prescribed on a temporary basis, either as a "bridge therapy" to get relief while awaiting for DMARD therapy to take effect, or for patients unable to tolerate NSAIDs. Corticosteroid use always requires careful supervision by a physician, and corticosteroids must never be abruptly halted without your doctor's knowledge. Proper use of this drug requires ongoing monitoring, and if necessary, gradual discontinuation.

CHAPTER 4

A Revolution in Arthritis Treatment

The last half century prior to 1998 had seen few break-throughs in drug therapies for RA. In the 1930s, the big news was sulfa-based drugs like sulfasalazine, which contained both an anti-inflammatory and anti-bacterial component (some people believe that RA is triggered by an infection). Corticosteroids hit the scene in the 1940s, bringing about dramatic improvement in RA symptoms, but also causing serious side effects because of the toxicity of high doses.

Methotrexate was first introduced in the 1940s as a leukemia drug. It showed great promise in the 1980s when it became widely used in RA treatment, and is still considered the gold standard against which all new medicines for RA are measured.

As science advanced in the 1980s and 1990s, particularly in the area of autoimmune disorders, so did research among pharmaceutical companies. The result was the long-awaited development of new agents for treating arthritis in general and

RA specifically. Among the arthritis drugs that have been made available in the United States since 1998 are:

- Celebrex® (celecoxib)
- Vioxx® (rofecoxib)
- Bextra® (valdecoxib)
- Mobic® (meloxicam)
- Arava® (leflunomide)
- Kineret® (anakinra)
- Enbrel® (etanercept)
- Remicade® (infliximab)
- Humira™ (adalimumab)

THE COX-2 INHIBITORS: CELEBREX®, VIOXX® AND BEXTRA®

In the late 1990s, two new drugs for arthritis — Celebrex® (celecoxib) and Vioxx® (rofecoxib) — were introduced in the U.S. These two medicines represented a completely new category of drugs for arthritis called cyclooxygenase-2 (COX-2) inhibitors. Bextra® (valdecoxib) is a similar agent that was introduced in 2002. The big news with these drugs was that they were as effective as traditional NSAIDs in treating inflammation, but were less likely to cause troublesome stomach-related side effects.

How COX-2 Inhibitors Work

COX-2 inhibitors are a novel addition to the medicines used to treat inflammation. To appreciate just how remarkable these drugs are, it is important to understand how NSAIDs work.

NSAIDs, such as Aleve® (naproxen) and Advil® or Motrin® (ibuprofen), inhibit enzymes called cyclooxygenase (COX). There are two types of COX enzymes: COX-1 and COX-2.

COX-1 enzymes are normally present in many tissues of the body and are beneficial in a number of ways, including protecting the lining of the stomach, and maintaining normal platelet function. (Platelets are the component of blood responsible for clotting.)

COX-2 enzymes contribute to the pain and swelling associated with arthritis and other conditions. Traditional NSAIDs inhibit both the COX-1 enzymes as well as the COX-2 enzymes.

COX-2 inhibitors reduce pain and inflammation but are less likely to cause the stomach-related side effects that are associated with traditional NSAIDs. These unwanted side effects include heartburn, ulcers and bleeding.

Safety Profile of COX-2 Inhibitors

COX-2 inhibitors are generally considered safe and effective for most people. However, a review[7] of two large post-marketing[8] clinical studies involving Celebrex® and Vioxx® was published in the *Journal of the American Medical Association*. The report showed that there may be an increased risk of heart attack in patients taking these COX-2 inhibitors. This is particularly true with Vioxx®, which was associated

---

7   Mukherjee D, Nissen SE, Topol EJ. Risk of cardiovascular events associated with selective COX-2 inhibitors. *JAMA* 2001;286(8):954-958.

8   "Post-marketing" is a term used to describe events that occur after the drug has been approved by the FDA for commercial marketing.

with a higher incidence of cardiovascular events in clinical studies than was Celebrex® or Bextra®. Although the significance of this finding is not clear, people identified to be at risk for heart attack should use COX-2 inhibitors with caution. Your physician may recommend the addition of baby aspirin to your regular medication regimen, but the aspirin may decrease the gastrointestinal protection offered by the COX-2 inhibitor.

The use of COX-2 inhibitors during pregnancy has not been studied. If you are pregnant or nursing you should not begin COX-2 inhibitor therapy. If you are trying to conceive and are taking a COX-2 inhibitor, talk with your doctor. A traditional NSAID may be preferred.

Side Effects of COX-2 Inhibitors

COX-2 inhibitors have been used safely and successfully by patients around the world. Still these drugs may cause other side effects seen with conventional NSAIDs. For these reasons, the FDA requires that manufacturers of COX-2 inhibitors report the same warnings about side effects as NSAIDs currently on the market. These potential side effects include, but are not limited to:

- Gastrointestinal symptoms, such as stomach ulcers, with or without bleeding; mouth ulcers, indigestion and abnormal liver function tests
- Renal problems, such as kidney damage
- Edema (swelling)
- Rash; on rare occasions, a life-threatening, blister-like rash (Stevens-Johnson syndrome) may develop

- Blood abnormalities, such as a decrease in blood counts, which increases the risk of bleeding or infection
- Photosensitivity; patients taking COX-2 inhibitors may develop a rash from sun exposure, and should avoid direct sunlight, or use precautions such as a sunscreen or hat
- Life-threatening allergic reactions in people with a history of asthma and nasal polyps
- Thrombotic events, including heart attack, stroke, and blood clots

Potential Drug Interactions With COX-2 Inhibitors

Taking a COX-2 inhibitor or a conventional NSAID with other medications can sometimes cause unwanted side effects. Taking multiple medications can also sometimes cause unwanted side effects. Although you should always check with your physician before beginning a COX-2 inhibitor, there are several potential drug interactions. These include, but are not limited to:

- Blood pressure and heart medications. This includes ACE inhibitors, such as Capoten® (captopril), Vasotec® (enalapril) and others. COX-2 inhibitors may have a two-fold effect when used in combination with ACE inhibitor therapy. First, the drug may reduce the benefit of ACE inhibitor therapy, resulting in higher blood pressure readings. It may also increase the risk of side effects from the combination, including decreasing kidney function or elevating potassium levels. Be sure to talk with your doctor if you take both a COX-2 inhibitor and blood pressure or heart medication.

- Dyazide® (triamterene/hydrochlorothiazide combination). Triamterene, in combination with a COX-2 inhibitor, can occasionally cause dangerously high levels of potassium in the blood, or decreased kidney function.

- Aspirin. The combination of aspirin and a COX-2 inhibitor may lessen the COX-2 inhibitor's stomach-protective qualities and increase the risk of stomach ulcers or other complications. On the other hand, aspirin may reduce the risk of thrombotic events, such as heart attack, stroke or blood clots. Consult with your physician before taking aspirin with a COX-2 inhibitor.

- Coumadin® (warfarin). The combination of a COX-2 inhibitor and warfarin may increase prothrombin (clotting) time and the risk of bleeding. Close monitoring is recommended.

Celebrex® (Celecoxib)

Celebrex® is FDA-approved for the treatment of rheumatoid arthritis (RA) and osteoarthritis. Introduced in the United States in the spring of 1999, it was the first COX-2 inhibitor on the market. It is taken once or twice a day to reduce pain and swelling.

Dosage and regimen. Celebrex® is taken in pill form. For RA, Celebrex® is taken in a 100 mg or 200 mg dosage twice a day. For osteoarthritis, it can be administered as 100 mg twice a day, or 200 mg in a single daily dosage. Celebrex® can be taken with or without food.

Contraindications. Celebrex® has a sulfa component, which may cause an allergic reaction in patients with a sensitivity to sulfa or sulfa-based drugs. Celebrex® can also aggravate asthma. It should not be given to patients who have experienced asthma, urticaria, or allergic-type reactions after taking aspirin or other NSAIDs. Severe, but rarely fatal allergic, anaphylactic-like reactions to NSAIDs have been reported in such patients. Nor should Celebrex® be used if you have a significant kidney, liver or blood disorder.

Vioxx® (Rofecoxib)

Vioxx® received FDA clearance in the summer of 1999, several months after Celebrex® was introduced. Vioxx® is approved to treat rheumatoid arthritis and osteoarthritis.

Vioxx® is similar to Celebrex® in many ways. It is used to treat pain and swelling, and as a COX-2 inhibitor, it is more protective of the stomach than conventional NSAIDs. It is also expensive as compared to standard NSAIDs, so Vioxx® may be reserved for those who are most at risk for gastrointestinal problems, e.g., people older than 65, those who smoke or have a history of an ulcer.

One important difference between this drug and the other COX-2 inhibitors is that Vioxx® does not contain a sulfa component. So it may be prescribed instead of Celebrex® or Bextra® (discussed later in this chapter) for people with a sensitivity to sulfa.

Dosage and regimen. Vioxx® is available both in pill and liquid form. It is prescribed at a dosage of 12.5 mg to

25 mg in a single daily dosage. A single daily 50 mg dosage of Vioxx® is FDA-approved for acute pain in osteoarthritis, but use of this higher dosage for prolonged periods (five days or more) has not been studied. Vioxx® can be taken with or without food.

Contraindications. Vioxx® should not be given to patients who have experienced asthma, urticaria, or allergic-type reactions after taking aspirin or other NSAIDs. Severe, but rarely fatal allergic, anaphylactic-like reactions to NSAIDs have been reported in such patients. Nor should Vioxx® be used if you have a significant kidney, liver or blood disorder.

Bextra® (Valdecoxib)

Bextra® is the newest of the COX-2 inhibitors. It was introduced in the United States in 2002, and is approved for both osteoarthritis and RA, as well as menstrual cramping.

Bextra® is generally well tolerated. Common side effects are headache, abdominal pain, nausea, diarrhea and upper respiratory infection. In clinical studies, there were several reports of serious stomach bleeding and serious skin reactions (e.g., Stevens-Johnson syndrome), although these reactions were rare.

Dosage and regimen. Bextra® is available only in pill form. For OA and RA, it is prescribed at a dosage of 10 mg in a single daily dosage. For best results, the drug should be taken on a consistent daily basis, not just for flare-ups. Bextra® can be taken with or without food.

Contraindications. Like Celebrex®, Bextra® has a sulfa component, which may cause an allergic reaction in patients with a sensitivity to sulfa or sulfa-based drugs. Bextra® can also aggravate asthma. It should not be given to patients who have experienced asthma, urticaria, or allergic-type reactions after taking aspirin or other NSAIDs. Severe, but rarely fatal allergic, anaphylactic-like reactions to NSAIDs have been reported in such patients.

A NEW AND IMPROVED NSAID: MOBIC®

Mobic® (meloxicam) is a new type of NSAID that works like a traditional NSAID with some of the properties of COX-2 inhibitors. Mobic® received FDA approval in 2000 to treat pain and inflammation in osteoarthritis. In Europe, Mobic® is also used to treat RA and ankylosing spondylitis, although it is not FDA-cleared for these applications in the United States.

How Mobic® (Meloxicam) Works

Mobic® has some of the protective gastrointestinal benefits of COX-2 inhibitors with some of the detriments of older-type NSAIDs. The drug shows selectivity in blocking the action of harmful COX-2 enzymes that contribute to pain and inflammation in conditions like arthritis. Mobic® also blocks the action of COX-1 enzymes, although to a lesser extent than traditional NSAIDs. So even though Mobic® works like a COX-2 inhibitor, it may be less protective of the stomach if you take more than 7.5 mg daily.

General Information About Mobic®

Dosage and regimen. Mobic® is administered in tablet form. It is prescribed at a dosage of 7.5 to 15 mg once daily. Mobic® can be taken with or without food.

Contraindications. Mobic® is contraindicated in patients with known hypersensitivity to the drug. It should not be given to patients who have experienced asthma, urticaria, or allergic-type reactions after taking aspirin or other NSAIDs. Severe, but rarely fatal allergic, anaphylactic-like reactions to NSAIDs have been reported in such patients.

Safety profile. Mobic® has been shown to be safe and effective in clinical studies. These studies showed that Mobic® 7.5 mg or 15 mg daily was more effective than placebo[9] in treating the signs and symptoms of osteoarthritis.

Side effects and warnings. In clinical studies, Mobic® caused gastrointestinal upset in 10 to 20 percent of patients. The most common stomach-related side effects were diarrhea, upset stomach and nausea.

The effect of Mobic® in pregnancy has not been studied. Women who are pregnant or nursing should not begin this drug. Women who are planning to become pregnant should discuss their situation with their physician before using this drug.

---

9   The term "placebo" refers to a dummy medication, such as a sugar pill, that has no specific pharmacologic action against the patient's illness or complaint.

Potential drug interactions. Taking Mobic® with other medications can cause unwanted side effects. Your pharmacist is a good source of information about potential drug interactions between Mobic® and other medications, including:

- Blood pressure and heart medications. This includes ACE inhibitors, such as Capoten® (captopril), Vasotec® (enalapril) and others. Mobic® may slightly reduce the antihypertensive benefit of ACE inhibitor therapy, resulting in higher blood pressure readings.

- Dyazide® (triamterene/hydrochlorothiazide combination). The use of Mobic® with this drug can occasionally cause dangerously high levels of potassium in the blood, or decreased kidney function.

- Aspirin. The combination of aspirin and Mobic® may increase the risk of stomach ulcers or other complications. On the other hand, aspirin may reduce the risk of thrombotic events, such as heart attack, stroke or blood clots. Talk with your physician or pharmacist if you use both medications concurrently.

A NEW AND NOVEL DMARD: ARAVA®

Arava® (leflunomide) was introduced in the United States in September 1998. It is indicated in adults for the treatment of active rheumatoid arthritis to reduce signs and symptoms of the disease.

Arava® acts much like existing DMARDs to slow the progression of RA and inhibit structural damage as evidenced by joint erosions on x-ray. Arava® has also been shown to reduce joint pain and inflammation and to improve physical function. The drug is considered expensive when compared with existing DMARDs, and has benefits similar to what can be attained with methotrexate. However, when compared with other biologic DMARDs, Arava® can cost significantly less. A one-month supply is about a quarter of the cost of Kineret®, and a fraction of the cost of Enbrel®, Remicade® or Humira™.

How Arava® (Leflunomide) Works

Arava® works to decrease inflammation by inhibiting the formation of pyrimidines. Pyrimidines are needed for cellular growth. It is thought that blocking the production of pyrimidines also inhibits the growth of activated immune cells in the joint.

General Information About Arava®

Dosage and regimen. Arava® is given in pill form. It is available in 10 mg, 20 mg and 100 mg tablets. When therapy is started, Arava® is dosed at 100 mg once a day for up to three days. This initial "loading" is followed by a maintenance dose of 20 mg daily, or 10 mg if the drug is not well tolerated. Arava® can be taken with or without food.

The combination of Arava® with methotrexate is being studied in an attempt to get a better clinical result. The combination has been reported to be effective for some patients. At this time, however, there are limited data available regarding this combination of treatments.

Contraindications. Arava® should not be prescribed in patients with a history of alcohol abuse, cirrhosis, hepatitis B or C, other liver abnormalities, lung disease or a history of recurring infections. The drug should not be used in pregnant and nursing women; nor should it be prescribed for women of childbearing age unless reliable birth control is being used. Patients should avoid excessive alcohol use while taking Arava®.

Safety profile and precautions. In clinical studies leading to FDA approval, Arava® was shown to be safe and effective in improving signs and symptoms of RA and in slowing joint damage. Subsequent studies of the drug's impact on patients' health-related quality of life led to revised labeling that indicated the drug for improved physical function in RA. However, the drug has not been without controversy. In the past several years, the safety of Arava® has been widely debated, particularly with regard to liver toxicity and the risk of serious infection.

There is no question that Arava® is an effective drug for RA, but like so many powerful anti-rheumatic agents, it should be used with caution in certain situations.

Long half-life. It is important to know that Arava® has a very long half-life. This means that it stays in your body for a long period of time. A long half-life is beneficial if the drug works for you. However, if you decide to discontinue the drug for any reason, it can take up to two years to rid your body of this drug. In these situations, your doctor will prescribe a drug called Questran® (cholestyramine) to speed up the process of eliminating the drug from your body.

Arava® and liver function. Post-marketing data indicated that Arava® may be linked to an increased risk of liver damage. Reports of patients with serious or fatal liver damage while taking leflunomide were widely reported in the media. The controversy caused a national patient advocacy group to petition the FDA to withdraw the drug from the market.

In a subsequent year-long review of data from six large studies involving more than 13,000 patients treated with Arava®, the Arthritis Advisory Committee of the FDA determined that "there was no unexpected life-threatening or serious clinically significant liver disease associated with Arava® in a way that could not be explained by multiple other factors, including simultaneous use of methotrexate without appropriate monitoring, alcohol intake, and simultaneous exposure to several other hepatotoxins."[10]

Based on this data, the FDA advisory committee agreed that "the incidence of patients who developed acute liver failure with Arava® was less than 1 in 50,000. This is similar to the risk of liver failure in patients taking methotrexate."

To address patient and physician concerns about liver toxicity, Arava's manufacturer addressed a letter[11] to physicians in October 2003. The letter informed physicians that rare, serious hepatic injury, including cases with a fatal outcome, had been reported in worldwide post-marketing

---

10 Fox RI, Kavanaugh A, Kremer J, et al. Rheumatoid arthritis: surveying the therapeutic horizon. *Med Crossfire.* 2003;4(9).

11 Aventis Pharmaceuticals. Important prescribing information (letter to physicians). October 2003. Available at www.fda.gov/medwatch/SAFETY/2003/safety03.htm#arava. Accessed January 17, 2004.

experience with the drug. Most of these incidences occurred within six months of therapy, and involved patients with multiple risk factors for liver toxicity.

As a result, Arava® should be used with caution if you are taking other medications that can also be toxic to the liver. These medications include, but are not limited to, methotrexate, NSAIDs, Celebrex®, Vioxx®, Bextra® and many others. As mentioned earlier, it is also important to avoid alcohol while taking Arava®. Arava® should not be prescribed if you have a history of alcohol abuse, cirrhosis, hepatitis B or C, other liver abnormalities.

Regular lab tests are recommended throughout Arava® therapy to monitor liver function. Testing is usually done at the start of therapy, and then monthly for at least six months. If the drug is well tolerated with no sign of liver toxicity, testing may decrease to once every two months. If liver enzymes increase beyond the normal range, the physician may opt to decrease the dose or discontinue the therapy. Due to the risk of bone marrow toxicity, complete blood counts (CBCs) should be checked at similar intervals.

Arava® and the respiratory system. There have been reports of several deaths due to interstitial pneumonia among Arava® users. Leflunomide's manufacturer advises additional precautions when prescribing the medication for patients with previous or existing lung conditions, or among those who show respiratory signs such as coughing after starting on the drug.

Arava® and serious infection. The October 2003 letter[12] sent to physicians by Arava's manufacturer also acknowledged rare reports of severe infection, including life-threatening or fatal sepsis, during post-marketing experience with the drug. In most of these cases, the patients were undergoing additional immunosuppressive therapy or had another medical condition in addition to rheumatoid disease that predisposed them to serious infection.

For this reason, if you have any sign or symptom of infection during Arava® therapy, you should call your doctor. It may be necessary to discontinue the therapy until the infection clears.

Arava®, fertility and pregnancy. Arava® has not been studied in pregnant humans, but the drug caused serious birth defects in animal studies. Due to the potential risk of injury to the developing fetus, Arava® should not be used by women of childbearing age who are sexually active, unless reliable birth control is being used. In fact, your physician may recommend that you use two forms of reliable birth control. Nor should the drug be used in children. Arava® has not been studied in women who are breastfeeding, and should not be used by nursing mothers. Nor should you begin on Arava® if you are pregnant or are considering pregnancy. Contact your physician immediately if you become pregnant, your period is late, or you want to begin trying to conceive. Your doctor will likely prescribe Questran® (cholestyramine) to eliminate Arava®

---

12 Aventis Pharmaceuticals. Important prescribing information (letter to physicians). October 2003. Available at www.fda.gov/medwatch/SAFETY/2003/safety03.htm#arava. Accessed January 17, 2004.

completely from your system, and recommend that you wait one full menstrual cycle before trying to conceive.

There is currently no evidence that Arava® affects fertility in men or women. Nor do available data suggest that Arava® increases the risk of male-mediated fetal damage. To minimize this potential risk, men wanting to father a baby should discontinue Arava® and consult their doctor. He/she will likely prescribe Questran® (cholestyramine) and advise waiting at least three months before trying to conceive.

Arava® and cancer. In animal studies, Arava® was associated with an increased risk of cancer. However there has not been sufficient evidence to date to link Arava® with malignancies in humans.

Side effects. Arava® can cause a variety of unwanted side effects. These include, but are not limited to:

- Gastrointestinal symptoms, including stomach discomfort, mouth ulcers, nausea, weight loss and diarrhea
- Skin problems, including rash or hair loss
- Neurological symptoms, such as dizziness, headache and numbness in any area of the body

Potential drug interactions. As mentioned earlier, you should be cautious about combining Arava® therapy with other medications that may also cause liver toxicity. Use of any other RA drug with Arava® has not been studied and should be considered experimental.

THE BIOLOGIC DMARDS: KINERET®, ENBREL®, REMICADE® AND HUMIRA™

The introduction of Enbrel® in 1998 hailed the arrival of an entirely new and vitally important category of drug to treat rheumatoid arthritis (RA) . This category of drugs is called "biologic DMARDs." Biologic DMARDs differ from other arthritis drugs in a very significant way. They act directly and specifically on the immune system to bring about relief from inflammation and swelling.

Kineret® (Anakinra)

Kineret® was approved for RA by the FDA in late 2001. It is used in patients with moderate to severe RA who have not responded to one or more conventional DMARDs. The drug is used to relieve signs and symptoms of the disease, as well as slow the progression of joint damage.

How Kineret® works. Kineret® is a biologic DMARD, meaning that it targets a specific biologic process that is implicated in rheumatoid arthritis. More specifically, Kineret® is a type of biologic DMARD called an interleukin-1 receptor antagonist (IL-1 RA). The drug works by neutralizing a cytokine called IL-1. Cytokines are the secreted products of activated immune cells. Cytokines such as IL-1 and TNF are the primary drivers of inflammation and damage in RA.

Dosage and regimen. Kineret® is given daily by subcutaneous injection. The standard dosage is 100 mg daily. The drug is provided in pre-filled syringes, and should be kept refrigerated until ready for use. The drug should then be brought to room temperature before injecting it. Kineret® may be used alone or in combination with methotrexate. Your doctor can supply you with a free automatic injector device if you need assistance with daily self injection.

Contraindications. Kineret® is contraindicated in people with a known allergy to Kineret® or its components. The drug is manufactured with recombinant DNA technology that uses an *E. coli* bacterial expression system. For this reason, Kineret® should not be used in people with a known sensitivity to *E. coli*-derived proteins.

Safety profile. In a number of clinical trials involving nearly 3,000 patients, approximately 40 percent of patients showed at least moderate improvement with Kineret®. The drug has also demonstrated a reduction in the progression of joint damage (as seen on x-ray) after 24 and 48 weeks of therapy.[13]

The long-term risks and benefits of Kineret® have not been evaluated, so long-term safety has not been established. Kineret® has not been studied in pregnant or nursing women. Although the drug did not cause birth defects in animal studies, the risks of Kineret® use in women who are pregnant, nursing or trying to conceive are unknown.

Side effects and warnings. Kineret® is generally well tolerated. The most common side effect is an injection site reaction, characterized by redness, inflammation or pain at

13 Cohen SB, Rubbert A. Bringing the clinical experience with anakinra to the patient. *Rheumatology.* 2003;42(Suppl.2):ii36-ii40.

the injection site. The reaction is typically mild and usually goes away after the first month of therapy.

Other side effects may include, but are not limited to: headache, diarrhea, flu-like symptoms, abdominal pain and rash.

Kineret® may cause a drop in white blood cell count, which may increase the risk of developing a serious infection, such as pneumonia. This risk is even greater in patients with asthma or chronic obstructive pulmonary disease (COPD). Thus, Kineret® should be used with caution if you have either condition.

In a small clinical study, patients who combined Kineret® therapy with a TNF blocker (such as Enbrel®) had lower white blood cell counts, and serious infections developed in 4 of 58 patients. As a result, Kineret® should not be used in combination with any other TNF inhibitor.

Potential drug interactions. There is limited experience with concomitant use of Kineret® and other drugs, and there are no known drug interactions at this time. Consult your physician or pharmacist if you have any questions about using Kineret® while taking other medications.

TNF Antagonists: Enbrel® (Etanercept), Remicade® (Infliximab) and Humira™ (Adalimumab)

In 1998, a new category of drugs to treat RA was introduced in the United States. Called "TNF blockers", "TNF inhibitors," "anti-TNF agents" or "TNF antagonists," this treatment was the first therapy to target tumor necrosis factor

(TNF). TNF is a biologic substance (called a cytokine) that has been implicated in the joint damage associated with rheumatoid arthritis.

There are currently three TNF blockers available in the United States — Enbrel® (etanercept), Humira™ (adalimumab), and Remicade® (infliximab). To say that these drugs have improved the lives of many arthritis patients might be considered an understatement. For some, these drugs are nothing short of a miracle.

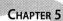

CHAPTER 5

TNF Blockers: The Arthritis Miracle

Victoria Archer vaguely recalls the first time she heard about TNF blockers. The news came one October morning in 1994 via her father-in-law, who phoned to tell her about an article he had just read in *USA Today*. An exciting new drug therapy for rheumatoid arthritis was in development and showing remarkable results in clinical trials. Victoria thanked him for the news, then promptly put it out of her mind. "After all," she says, "there are always new treatments in development. But I've had RA since 1974. A new treatment always begs the question, 'Will it be available in time to help me?'"

Nine years later, Victoria would learn the answer to her hypothetical question. In 2003, nearly 30 years after she was first diagnosed with rheumatoid arthritis, that answer was a resounding, "Yes!"

THE LONG-AWAITED MIRACLE FOR ARTHRITIS

The long-awaited breakthrough for arthritis is a category of drugs called "tumor necrosis factor alpha antagonists." This cumbersome name is often shortened to "TNF-α blockers," or even more simply, "TNF blockers." These TNF-blocking drugs have many names, all of which are used interchangeably throughout this book:

- Anti-TNF compound
- Anti-TNF therapy
- TNF antagonist
- TNF-alpha antagonist

- TNF-α antagonist
- TNF blocker
- TNF-blocking therapy
- TNF inhibitor

The first of the TNF blockers — Enbrel® — was introduced in the United States in November 1998. Others were subsequently approved in 1999 and 2002. What makes these drugs so revolutionary, especially when compared with conventional RA drugs, is that they inhibit the action of a biologic substance called the tumor necrosis factor (TNF).

THE TUMOR NECROSIS FACTOR (TNF)

Tumor necrosis factor is a substance produced naturally by your immune system. It is a important type of protein, called a cytokine, that acts as a chemical messenger between cells. In small amounts, TNF is a good thing. It is one of several cytokines[14] that helps to promote normal inflammatory and immune responses. However, in excess amounts, TNF can wreak havoc on your body's immune response.

---

14 There are a number of cytokines that play a role in the inflammatory response and are being investigated as potential treatments in autoimmune diseases. In addition to TNF-α and TNF-β, there are interleukin-1 (IL-1), interleukin-2 (IL-2) and many others.

TNF and the Normal Immune Response

When an infection or another event kicks your immune system into action, TNF begins its work at the cellular level. It attaches to other chemical receptors, called TNF receptors, that are located on the surface of cells.

There are two different TNF receptors. The first is a 55-kilodalton protein, dubbed "p55." (A kilodalton is a measure of a molecule's size.) The other is a 75-kilodalton protein known as "p75." When TNF binds to either of these two receptors, a chemical reaction occurs. The result of this chemical reaction is inflammation, which is the normal response of a healthy immune system.

A Brief History of TNF

The effect of the tumor necrosis factor was first observed in 1893 by William B. Coley, M.D. Dr. Coley, a surgeon at Memorial Hospital in New York City (now Memorial Sloan-Kettering Cancer Center), was reviewing case information about patients with bone cancer. He noticed that patients who developed a bacterial infection after surgery seemed to have higher rates of cancer regression. In this selected patient population, cancerous bone tumors had a tendency to "necrose," meaning that the cancerous cells died off and the tumors shrank.

Dr. Coley theorized that the bacterial infection must somehow stimulate the immune system, causing it to fight harder against the cancer cells. He hoped that he might be able to effect a cure based on this theory. He produced extracts of specific bacterial cultures, and administered them by injection to cancer patients. In doing so, Dr. Coley unknowingly launched the field of immunotherapy.

Despite anecdotal reports of cancer regression associated with "Coley toxins," the approach was considered controversial and never gained widespread acceptance. The treatment was largely abandoned in favor of cytotoxic radiotherapy, an anti-cancer treatment that was in development at the same time.

It would take more than 75 years before researchers would turn their attention back to Coley's promising observations. In 1975, clinical researchers determined that bacterial endotox-ins contained in Coley toxins stimulated immune cells to secrete a substance that causes an anti-tumor reaction. By 1985, researchers had demonstrated that this substance had a direct necrotic effect on tumor cells. And so this substance was named the "tumor necrosis factor."

TNF-α Versus TNF-β

Scientific advances in the 1980s and 1990s led to a better understanding of the tumor necrosis factor. Two forms of TNF have since been identified: tumor necrosis factor alpha (TNF-α) and tumor necrosis factor beta (TNF-β). TNF-α and TNF-β are both cytokines, which are proteins secreted by different types of cells that regulate the body's immune response. A primary difference between the two is that TNF-α is secreted by a type of white blood cell called a macrophage, while TNF-β is secreted by a type of white blood cell called a T-cell, specifi-cally the T helper cytotoxic cells.

The distinction is an important one, because scientists have discovered that people with rheumatoid arthritis produce an overabundance of TNF-α.[15] For reasons unknown, in RA the normal immune response goes awry, and stimulates the secretion of cytokines — and specifically TNF-α.

This triggers a series of severe inflammatory responses in what is called the "pro-inflammatory cytokine cascade." The release of TNF induces the production of other pro-inflammatory cytokines, which multiplies the effect of the immune response and causes joint inflammation, swelling, tenderness and pain. Over time, this hyper-immune response begins to attack once-healthy tissues. If left untreated, TNF-α can eventually destroy the joints and damage other organs.

TNF BLOCKERS FOR RA

When scientists realized the significant role that TNF-α plays in RA, they focused their research on developing anti-TNF agents to treat the disease. Their work has been very successful. Today, there are three TNF blockers available in the United States:

- Enbrel® (etanercept)
- Remicade® (infliximab)
- Humira™ (adalimumab)

All three of these drugs block TNF-α. Enbrel® also has an effect on TNF-β.

---

15 TNF-α is also implicated in psoriatic arthritis, ankylosing spondylitis, and juvenile chronic arthritis. Scientists now believe that both TNF-α and TNF-β may play a role in JCA.

Enbrel® (etanercept) was the first FDA-approved TNF antagonist available in the United States. It is approved for a broader range of indications than any other of the TNF blockers. Specifically, Enbrel® is approved for five indications: (1) to treat the signs and symptoms and delay structural damage in patients with early-stage RA; (2) moderate-to-severe RA; (3) psoriatic arthritis; (4) ankylosing spondylitis; and, (5) in children with polyarticular juvenile chronic arthritis who have not responded to DMARDs alone.

Remicade® (infliximab) is FDA-approved — in combination with methotrexate — for the treatment of rheumatoid arthritis in patients who have had an inadequate response to methotrexate alone. The drug is also approved for use in patients with Crohn's disease who have not responded to conventional therapy. (Crohn's disease is an inflammatory condition that affects the colon. Arthritis may also accompany this illness.)

Humira™ (adalimumab) is also FDA-approved for reducing the signs and symptoms of moderate to severe RA in people who have not responded to one or more DMARDs. It is the newest of the three TNF blockers, and was introduced in late 2002.

HOW TNF BLOCKERS WORK

TNF blockers help the body by "down-regulating" the high levels of TNF found in RA and other forms of inflammation. The drugs must be either injected or given intravenously. This "floods" the body with the anti-TNF agent. In the case of Enbrel®, the drug then acts as a sponge to remove excess

TNF-α molecules from the body. In the case of Remicade® and Humira™, the drug binds to excess TNF-α molecules in the body. This action changes their molecular structure and neutralizes their pro-inflammatory effect.

> 66 I feel fortunate to live at a time and in a place where so much research and development is being done on drug therapies like TNF blockers. When I first learned I had RA, I envisioned my life as not very pleasant over the long term. My quality of life is good now, due in large part to TNF blockers. 99
>
> — Sarah Olson, 56, started TNF blocker therapy for RA in February 2000

The results can be life-changing. TNF blockers substantially reduce inflammation, decrease the number of swollen and tender joints, prevent joint damage and fight the fatigue that is common with RA. Many patients talk about "feeling normal" again, and feel well enough to resume pleasurable activities they have avoided for years because of their unrelenting arthritis.

TNF blockers are also being studied as potential treatments for a wide range of medical conditions. These include uveitis (inflammation of the eye), asthma, Alzheimer's disease, vasculitis (inflammation of the blood vessels), cervical disc disease (a condition of the cervical spine) and sciatica (a painful condition affecting the lower back and legs). TNF blockers may also one day have an application in graft versus host disease to reduce rejection of organ transplants.

THE SCIENCE BEHIND THE ARTHRITIS MIRACLE

Enbrel®, Remicade® and Humira™ are all protein-based drugs. Remicade® and Humira™ are referred to as "IgG1 mono-clonal antibodies (mAb) specific for the human tumor necrosis factor." Enbrel® is described as a "recombinant p75-TNF receptor linked to the Fc portion of human IgG1."

A brief explanation may help to make sense of these complex scientific descriptions. The term "monoclonal antibodies" describes immunoglobulins (Ig) that are produced in the laboratory for a variety of medicinal purposes. Immunoglobulins are protein[16] molecules found in the blood that enable the body to recognize foreign proteins, such as a virus or bacteria.

Immunoglobulins are Y shaped. The end portions of the Y are called the "variable region." One arm of the Y contains a "heavy" chain of amino acids. The other arm contains a "light" chain of amino acids. This feature allows immunoglobulins to be highly variable, and therefore, specific for a particular antigen (foreign or harmful substance), such as TNF-α.

The stem of the Y plays an important role in the physiologic processes that neutralize or eliminate the antigen to which the Ig is specific. The molecular structure of the stem is identical in all antibodies of the same class, and is known as the "constant region."

---

16 Proteins are large molecules that are made up of amino acids. Proteins are often called the "building blocks of the body," and are responsible for most of the functions and much of the structure of the human body (and, in fact, all living things.)

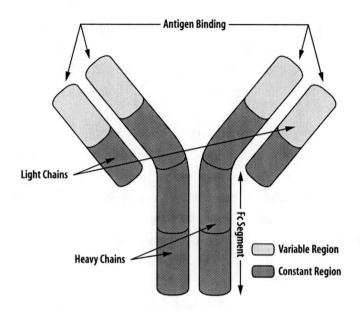

Structure of an immunoglobulin.

Scientists have identified nine immunoglobulins in five classes. The five classes are designated as IgA, IgD, IgE, IgG and IgM. In addition, IgA has two subclasses, IgA1 and IgA2. IgG has four subclasses, IgG1, IgG2, IgG3 and IgG4.

Each type of immunoglobulin plays a different role in defending the body against foreign proteins. IgG1 is the major immunoglobulin found in the blood. IgG1 is also able to enter other cellular structures, where it locates and captures antigens, and facilitates their removal by other cells in the immune system. TNF antagonists are based on IgG1.

HOW TNF BLOCKERS ARE MADE

Enbrel®, Remicade® and Humira™ are manufactured using recombinant methods. This means that the medications are genetically engineered in the laboratory using DNA technology. Making these biotech compounds is quite complex, time-consuming and expensive compared with conventional pharmaceutical compounds.

Manufacturing conventional medications, which are called "small molecule drugs," is a relatively straightforward process. The process involves heating and cooling chemical compounds to isolate the active ingredient. Dry, inactive ingredients, such as coloring and flavoring agents, are added. After testing for quality, the compound is compressed into pills or tablets and packaged. Large batches can be manufactured in a few weeks.

Biotech medications require a completely different manufacturing methodology. Unlike conventional medications that are absorbed in the bloodstream and cause a chemical reaction that spreads through the body, biotech drugs are man-made versions of natural proteins that target a specific biologic process involved in the disease process. Making copies of these natural proteins is much more complex than simply mixing and processing chemical compounds. Producing these compounds requires living cells — in a word, biology.

Enbrel® and Remicade® use living organisms to produce or "express" the proteins that are the basis of TNF antagonist treatment. The selected cell type is chosen for its safety and ability to express proteins that are similar in structure to proteins found naturally in the body.

In the case of Enbrel®, human DNA is introduced into Chinese hamster ovary cells. These ovarian cells act as living factories to manufacture a genetically engineered protein. The resulting protein is an exact replica of the p75-TNF receptor fused to a specific area of the IgG1 molecule's constant region known as the Fc segment.

Remicade® uses a combination of human and mouse proteins to create a hybrid IgG1 protein that is known as a "chimeric" monoclonal antibody. Humira™ is produced from fully human proteins using "phage display" technology. This process uses bacteriophages[17] to produce or "display" human monoclonal antibodies on their surface. Humira™ is the first biologic drug to use fully human proteins.

Producing man-made IgG1 is an intricate process.[18] As described in an article by business reporter Luke Timmerman in the *Seattle Times,* the cells are placed in large stainless-steel vats that are filled with a nutrient broth. The broth supplies the necessary vitamins, minerals and amino acids required for the cells' survival and growth. The cells and broth are maintained under tightly-controlled environmental parameters, including temperature, oxygen and acidity. Under ideal conditions, the cells produce the IgG1 protein that is the basis of TNF antagonist therapy. After a period of time, the cellular mix is harvested, filtered, then purified to inactivate viruses and isolate the IgG1 protein. The protein is tested extensively to ensure its purity before it is readied for distribution. Refrigeration is required to preserve the proteins.

---

17 Bacteriophages are viruses that infect bacteria but are harmless to humans.

18 Timmerman L. Biology calls shots in making a drug (part 2 of 3). *Seattle Times.* April 29, 2002. Available at www.seattletimes.com. Accessed February 28, 2004.

THE LONG-TERM PROMISE — AND RISKS — OF TNF BLOCKERS

In multiple clinical studies[19] involving tens of thousands of arthritis patients, TNF blockers produced noticeable improvement in at least 2 of every 3 patients. This success rate held true regardless of which TNF blocker was used.

What is most remarkable about this statistic is that the vast majority of patients in these early clinical trials had to have failed all existing treatments in order to qualify for the clinical trial. A 42-73 percent[20] success rate in the face of such a stubborn disease state is very encouraging, indeed.

> **66** What do you want from your life? What do you want to do each day? If you want more from your life or your current therapy is giving you problems, ask about TNF blockers. **99**
>
> — Joy Hollingsworth, 42, started TNF blocker therapy for RA in November 1999

The statistic also reveals an important point about TNF therapy. The lack of benefit or development of a bothersome side effect with one anti-TNF drug does not automatically preclude success with the other two.

Another positive finding both in clinical trials and in real-world practice is that side effects with TNF blockers are, in

---

19 Because all three TNF blockers work similarly, it is not unreasonable to draw broad conclusions about the entire class of drugs based on the outcome[s] of individual large, well-designed, placebo-controlled clinical trials that examine one or another of these therapies.

20 Personal correspondence between the authors and John J. Cush, M.D. March 30, 2004.

most cases, relatively minor. More significantly, among patients who have been on a TNF blocker for several years or more, the benefits appear to be long-lasting.

Even so, anti-TNF therapy is not without risks. Serious side effects can occur. About 1 in 1,000 patients will experience a serious adverse event with TNF blockers.[21] Vigilance and monitoring are the keys to minimizing the potential risks associated with these drugs. Following is a list of precautions and possible adverse side effects that you should be aware of with TNF antagonists.

TNF Blockers and Injection Site Reactions

The most common side effect with anti-TNF therapy is a mild injection or infusion site reaction (ISR). ISRs are characterized by redness, swelling and/or itching at the site where the drug is injected or infused. Less than one-third of all patients experience ISRs. However, fewer than 5 percent of patients discontinue the therapy because of the reaction.[22] ISRs tend to be mild to moderate in severity, are primarily seen in the first month of therapy, and become less bothersome over time.

TNF Blockers and Infection

TNF inhibitors are immunosuppressive. Not surprisingly, clinical studies indicate that people taking TNF blockers have an increased risk of developing infections, and infection is the

---

21 Cush, JJ. Safety of New Biologic Therapies in Rheumatoid Arthritis. *Bull Rheum Dis.* 2003;52(8).

22 Ibid.

second most common side effect of anti-TNF therapy. In clinical trials, upper respiratory infection, such as sinusitis, occurred
in about 1 of every 3 patients. But these infections also
occurred at nearly the same rate in patients taking placebo.

While most of these infections are relatively minor, there
are reports of patients who have developed serious infections.
Some of these infections were fatal.

In initial clinical studies that led to FDA approval of
Enbrel® and Remicade®, the incidence of serious infection was
infrequent. But in post-approval usage, serious infections,
including bacterial infections, tuberculosis and opportunistic
infections[23], have been reported with all three TNF blockers.

As a result, the latest TNF blocker to be approved by the
FDA — Humira™ — was scrutinized closely during pre-
approval clinical trials for the risk of serious infections versus
placebo. These trials showed that there was a increased incidence of serious and opportunistic infection among the
anti-TNF therapy group: 0.04 percent versus 0.02 percent for
placebo. An equally important finding was that these patients
were all treated promptly and appropriately, and their infections did not progress.

It is also important to note that your risk of developing a
serious infection while using a TNF blocker may increase if
you have a condition that predisposes you to infection.
Tuberculosis has been diagnosed in a small but increased per-

23 An opportunistic infection is one that typically occurs in people with an
immunosuppressive condition that causes a weakened immune system.

centage of patients who have been on TNF antagonists. Most of these infections involved patients living in Europe and other countries where tuberculosis is a more common infectious problem than in North America. Nonetheless, those most at risk for tuberculosis or another opportunistic infection while taking a TNF blocker include:

- People who have lived in endemic regions such as Europe
- Recent immigrants from areas of the world with high rates of tuberculosis or another opportunistic infection
- People who take prednisone regularly
- People who have been exposed to tuberculosis
- Intravenous drug users

A tuberculin skin test is recommended before anti-TNF treatment is started. Patients who have a positive skin test without signs or symptoms of active tuberculosis may be able to start therapy in conjunction with an anti-TB medication. Consultation with an infectious disease physician may be recommended.

Patients with uncontrolled diabetes, chronic kidney disease, lymphoma, silicosis, or HIV-positive status, are at increased risk for serious infections, and probably should not be started on TNF-blocking therapy.

TNF Blockers and the Development of Autoimmune Abnormalities

The use of TNF antagonists may result in the formation of autoantibodies that are commonly seen in lupus. About 5 to 50 percent of patients on anti-TNF therapy develop abnormal autoantibodies. The clinical significance of this finding is uncertain, but rarely do patients taking a TNF inhibitor develop lupus or another type of arthritis.

Lupus-like symptoms may include chest pain, and most commonly, a rash. While reports of lupus or lupus-like symptoms are rare, the symptoms usually improve once anti-TNF therapy is discontinued. To date, fewer than 30 patients have reported this complication.

In animal studies of lupus and demyelinating disease (e.g., multiple sclerosis), TNF has been shown to play a protective role against these illnesses. This observation may help to explain why a few patients being treated with TNF antagonists develop lupus, multiple sclerosis or related illnesses.

TNF Blockers and Blood Disorders

There is a slight risk of developing an abnormal blood condition while taking a TNF antagonist, which can increase your risk of developing a life-threatening infection. Several patients taking Enbrel® developed blood cell abnormalities. Some of these patients subsequently died. Similar effects are also a potential risk with other TNF antagonists.

As a result, if you have any sign or symptom of infection, including a cough, fever or shortness of breath; or signs of anemia, such as bruising, bleeding or paleness, you should notify your physician immediately. He or she can decide if you should temporarily discontinue the TNF blocker and/or begin antibiotic therapy.

TNF Blockers and Cancer (Malignancy)

There have been reports of patients developing lymphoma during anti-TNF therapy. Twenty-three of the first 6,300 patients prescribed TNF-blocking therapy in clinical trials developed lymphoma. The reports prompted the FDA to review post-marketing data regarding TNF blockers and cancer. In March 2003, the FDA's Arthritis Advisory Committee[24] concluded that a connection between TNF blockers and lymphoma was possible, but could not be established with certainty.[25] This was due to a number of reasons:

• The clinical trials that generated the data were small.

• Many of the patients involved in the clinical trials were taking TNF blockers in addition to other arthritis medications that are known to increase the risk of lymphoma.

• Rheumatoid arthritis by itself places patients at an increased risk for developing lymphoma, and this risk increases with the severity of the disease. Thus, people with severe RA are more likely to take TNF blockers — and these patients are already at higher risk for developing lymphoma compared with both the general population and other patients with milder forms of RA.

---

24 The commissioner of the FDA relies on formal advisory groups with specific knowledge in various disciplines to determine whether a medication or medical device can be considered safe and effective. The Arthritis Advisory Committee is one such group. The committee comprises authorities in the fields of arthritis, rheumatology, orthopedics, pain management, biostatistics and other specialties. They evaluate safety and efficacy data and make recommendations based on data collected during clinical trials as well as after the drug has been introduced in the U.S. (what is called the "post-marketing" phase).

25 Gibofsky A. TNF-alpha inhibitors and lymphoma: more data needed to assess risk. *New Developments in Rheumatic Diseases.* 2003;1(3):1-4.

So it is difficult to know if the incidence of lymphoma seen in these patients is attributable to the TNF blockers alone or the natural course of highly active RA.

- Although there were no cases of lymphoma in the placebo-treated patients, the FDA Advisory Committee noted that many of these patients were "cross-over" participants, meaning that they were switched from placebo to a TNF blocker after a period of time. As a result, there was a shorter follow-up period compared with patients who had been taking TNF blockers since the start of the trials. Thus, longer-term data on the placebo/cross-over patients that might have shown a similar incidence of lymphomas were not available for comparison.

- The incidence of lymphoma in the general population is increasing. Although patients taking TNF antagonists showed a higher incidence of lymphoma than the rate expected among the normal adult population (as calculated from the National Cancer Institute's SEER database, which uses data collected in 1992-1999), the risk is still considered relatively low. (SEER provides information about cancer incidence and survival in the United States.)

The challenge facing the FDA Advisory Committee is that the data were not able to demonstrate conclusively what portion of the new cases of lymphoma could be directly attributed to disease, what portion was attributable to the TNF blockers, and what portion was attributed to other factors, such as heredity or an environmental trigger, such as long-term exposure to a cancer-causing agent.

TNF Blockers and Central Nervous System Disorders

A rare but potential risk of TNF blockers is the development of a demyelinating disorder such as multiple sclerosis (MS), or worsening of pre-existing MS or optic neuritis. Although there have been no studies designed specifically to confirm or disprove a connection between MS and TNF blockers, the medical literature supports a possible connection. The general recommendation at this time is that anti-TNF therapy should not be prescribed for patients with MS or for those who have a history of optic neuritis or another demyelinating disorder. You should also notify your doctor if you develop MS or a related neurological disorder while taking a TNF antagonist.

TNF Blockers and Pregnancy

Enbrel®, Remicade® and Humira™ are all classified[26] as pregnancy risk category B. Essentially, this means that there are no data from large, well-designed clinical studies regarding the use of these drugs in pregnant or nursing women. So while Enbrel®, Remicade® and Humira™ are not specifically contraindicated in pregnancy, they probably should not be taken by patients who are pregnant or nursing unless clearly needed. Talk with your doctor if you plan to become pregnant, suspect

---

26 All drugs are assigned a pregnancy risk category (designated as category A, B, C, D or X) based on the level of risk the drug poses to the developing fetus. A drug's risk category is one of many factors considered when evaluating whether or not a drug is safe to use during pregnancy. Category A represents the least risk to the fetus, while category X indicates a drug that poses risk so great that it is contraindicated in women who are or may become pregnant. (Methotrexate is a category X drug.) Drugs assigned to category B, as is the case with Enbrel®, Remicade™ and Humira™, either: (1) did not cause damage to the fetus in animal trials, but there are no human clinical trials to either confirm or refute this; or (2) did cause damage to the fetus in animal studies, but did not cause damage to first-trimester fetuses in controlled human trials of the drug.

you are pregnant, or intend to nurse your infant. Sexually active men and women who will also be taking methotrexate during anti-TNF therapy need to use reliable birth control, because methotrexate — a pregnancy risk category X drug — has been associated with birth defects and miscarriages.

TNF Blockers and Cardiopulmonary Events

The effectiveness of TNF antagonists in RA raised the possibility that these drugs might also benefit people with congestive heart failure (CHF). Much like the role it plays in RA, TNF also affects both normal and abnormal cardiovascular function. Researchers sought to prove the theory that TNF blockers could be beneficial in CHF through several large, randomized, placebo-controlled studies. Unfortunately, they found the opposite to be true. Not only were TNF blockers not effective in treating CHF,[27] but in patients treated with Remicade® specifically, the drug was linked to a higher all-cause rate of mortality.[28] However, results from several more recent studies have generated mixed results concerning the influence of anti-TNF therapy on CHF. Until more definitive information is available, CHF-related adverse side effects should be considered a potential risk with all anti-TNF agents. Physicians should use caution when prescribing a TNF blocker in CHF patients and the drugs should be avoided in patients

27 Spencer-Green G, Warren MS, Whitmore J, et al. Effects of etanercept (Enbrel®) in patients with chronic heart failure: results of RENAISSANCE and RECOVER trials. Program and abstracts of the 66th Annual Scientific Meeting of the American College of Rheumatology; October 25-29, 2002; New Orleans, Louisiana. Abstract 1389.

28 Centocor, Inc. news release. Centocor places congestive heart failure clinical program on hold. October 22, 2001.

with significant[29] heart failure. CHF patients who take a TNF blocker should also be regularly monitored by a cardiologist.

In addition to congestive heart failure, TNF antagonists may pose an increased risk of serious cardiopulmonary side effects, such as chest pain, difficulty breathing, and low blood pressure, which can sometimes be life-threatening. This risk for these events was found to be low in clinical studies. Still, if you have a history of respiratory or cardio-vascular problems, your physician may recommend against anti-TNF therapy.

TNF Blockers and Other Possible Side Effects

As with all medications, TNF blockers can cause other unwanted adverse effects. There have been reports of such events, including, but not limited to, liver damage, kidney damage and vasculitis. For this reason, it is reasonable for your physician to order periodic laboratory studies such as a complete blood count (CBC) and blood chemistry as well as urinalysis to check for any changes or abnormalities while you are taking a TNF antagonist.

---

29 Heart failure is classified according to the severity of symptoms and to what extent patients are limited by symptoms during physical exertion. The most widely used classification system is called the New York Heart Association (NYHA) congestive heart failure (CHF) functional classification system, which assigns CHF patients to one of four categories (I, II, III, IV). Class I CHF is the least limiting, with few or no symptoms upon physical exertion. Class IV is severe CHF, where symptoms can occur with the slightest physical activity or even at rest. TNF blockers should be used with caution in people with class I or II CHF, and should be avoided in those with class III and IV.

A Final Word About the Risks of TNF Blockers

A presentation[30] by Joan M. Bathon, M.D.,[31] at a rheumatology symposium in October 2003 perhaps best summarizes the current state of knowledge regarding TNF antagonist therapy and how to navigate the unknown and potential risks of this treatment:

> "Some adverse events associated with chronic inhibition of TNF (e.g., opportunistic infections, including tuberculosis) can be predicted, based on the known physiologic roles of TNF. Other adverse events (e.g., congestive heart failure and multiple sclerosis) seem counterintuitive to the data generated from preclinical studies in animals. By studying the types of adverse events that occur with a new, highly specific therapy such as TNF antagonists, some insights can be obtained regarding the physiologic importance of the inhibited molecule.

> "Fortunately, TNF antagonists are highly effective in treating inflammatory diseases such as RA, and adverse events related to these agents are relatively rare. Nonetheless, screening for latent TB should be performed before beginning anti-TNF therapy, and TNF antagonists should be avoided in patients with uncontrolled CHF.

---

30 Bathon, JM. Clinical perspective on the physiologic and pathogenic roles of TNF (Part II). Presented at The Biologic Revolution in Rheumatoid Arthritis: How TNF Antagonists Have Optimized RA Treatment and Outcomes symposium, Orlando, Fla., October 25, 2003.

31 Dr. Bathon has received research support from Abbott Laboratories, Amgen Inc., and Centocor, Inc.

"...the risk of cancer or lymphoma in patients with RA treated with TNF antagonists appears to be consistent with the background rates in patients with RA as a whole. However, longer periods of observation and larger data bases will be needed to more accurately define this risk."

THE HIGH PRICE OF SCIENCE

The advanced science and DNA engineering that made TNF antagonist therapy possible also contributes to the high cost of this treatment. The retail cost for people without health insurance and/or prescription drug benefits ranges from $12,000 to over $60,000 per year.

Clearly, the cost is a barrier to treatment for some patients. It is also an ongoing concern for others, who worry about whether their health insurance plans will continue to provide coverage.

The issue of cost is one reason why it is too early to know if TNF blockers will one day soon become the standard of care for rheumatoid arthritis. Certainly, the benefits of TNF blockers are now being established and widely recognized, and a favorable cost/benefit ratio is beginning to take shape.

But methotrexate remains the gold standard of RA treatment. Based on the known efficacy, comparatively lower cost and long-term safety experience with methotrexate and MTX-combination therapies such as MTX/hydroxychloroquine and sulfasalazine, methotrexate compares favorably to TNF blockers. Methotrexate is also significantly more cost effective. This reality means that rheumatologists will likely continue to consider MTX as the gold-standard, first-line drug therapy for RA for some time to come.

Even so, TNF antagonists have made their mark on arthritis therapy — as they continue to restore both mobility and hope to thousands of arthritis patients around the world.

The next three chapters will take a closer look at each of the TNF antagonists currently available in the United States. You can judge for yourself the benefits and risks of these miracle drugs.

> 66 The only side effect I've had is stupidity. Sometimes I do more than I should because I forget I have arthritis. 99
>
> — Howard Weinberg, 60, began TNF blocker therapy for ankylosing spondylitis in May 1999

CHAPTER 6

Enbrel® (Etanercept)

Susan Holt was a sophomore at the University of Oklahoma when the doctors finally gave a name to the skin problems and severe joint pain that had sapped her energy and made it difficult to walk.

"Psoriatic arthritis," they told her.

"My life is over," the 22-year-old told herself.

Susan had no idea how wrong that assessment would be. But the road to realization wouldn't be easy. It started with anti-inflammatories, followed by gold, oral methotrexate, injectable methotrexate, then going without MTX during five years of infertility treatments. There were high points along the way, like her marriage to Jack in December 1996 — as well as the day she began Enbrel® therapy in January 2003.

Three weeks later, on February 25, 2003, she and Jack were on a plane to Virginia where they missed the birth of their adoptive daughter by just 10 minutes. But on this trip, it wasn't Susan's arthritis that slowed them down. An ice storm had delayed their flight out of Dallas. It was the last time anything would slow down this active 32-year-old mother, who is filled with optimism about her family's future.

"Having a child was so important to us. And knowing that a birth mother was entrusting us with her precious baby made it an even bigger responsibility because of my arthritis. Before Enbrel®, I worried about how I would care for the baby on my 'bad' days. Since starting on Enbrel®, I haven't had one yet."

ENBREL®: THE MOST WIDELY USED TNF BLOCKER

Enbrel® was the first TNF blocker available in the United States. When Enbrel® was introduced in November 1998, it represented the most significant breakthrough in RA therapy in two decades, offering millions of RA patients new hope for an improved quality of life. Enbrel's generic name is etanercept (pronounced ee-tan-er-sept).

Enbrel® is currently FDA-approved for the broadest range of indications of any TNF blocker. This landmark drug has earned additional approvals for new and expanded applications in nearly every year since it was first introduced in 1998.

Enbrel® is FDA-approved:

- To reduce the signs and symptoms of moderate to severe active RA in adults who have not responded adequately to one or more DMARDs (1998)
- To reduce the signs and symptoms in juvenile chronic arthritis (1999)
- As a first-line therapy for adults with early-stage RA (2000)

- To reduce the signs and symptoms of psoriatic arthritis (2002)
- To reduce the signs and symptoms of ankylosing spondylitis (2003)

ENBREL® AT A GLANCE

Generic name	Etanercept
Introduced	1998
Manufacturer	Amgen Inc.
Approved uses	Early-stage RA Moderate to severe RA Psoriatic arthritis Ankylosing spondylitis Polyarticular juvenile chronic arthritis
Delivery	Subcutaneous injection
Frequency	Once a week* or every 72-96 hours
Dosage	Adults: 25 mg per injection Children (ages 4-17): Max 0.8 mg/kg of body weight
Annual cost	$16,488

* Enbrel® was originally approved at a dosage of 25 mg every 72-96 hours (approx. twice weekly). A once-weekly 50 mg dosage was approved by the FDA in late 2003. The once-weekly treatment is administered via two 25-mg injections given on the same day.

IMPORTANT FACTS ABOUT ENBREL®

Enbrel® is supplied as a refrigerated white powder. The powder needs to be reconstituted (mixed) by the patient into a clear liquid and given as a 25 mg injection twice weekly. While some patients have reported significant improvement within one or two weeks of the first injection, most people respond within one month. Maximum benefit is typically attained within three months.

Of course, Enbrel® does not work for everyone who tries it. In practice, about 10 to 15 percent of participants did not respond to Enbrel® therapy. While Enbrel® has been shown to decrease joint damage from RA, it can not reverse existing joint deformities. Only people with active inflammation will potentially benefit from the drug. It will not help those who have damaged joints without active disease.

---

66 The difference between other drugs and Enbrel® is night and day. Other drugs are like taking an aspirin for pneumonia. Enbrel® is like taking a broad-spectrum antibiotic. It gets to the root of the problem and has a long-lasting effect. 99

— Carla Mason, 45, began Enbrel®
for RA in May 2000

HOW ENBREL® WORKS

Enbrel® is a recombinant human tumor necrosis factor receptor fusion protein. Enbrel® slows joint damage and the progression of RA in a novel way. The medication is administered by subcutaneous injection. The injection "floods" the body with Enbrel® molecules, which are man-made replicas of the p75 receptor fused to the Fc portion of the IgG1 molecule. (The p75 receptor is the cellular mechanism that TNF-alpha binds to. Refer to Chapter 5 for details about TNF and the science behind TNF blockers.) When these genetically engineered receptors are released into the body, they act as a sponge to remove a significant amount of TNF molecules from the joints and blood, before they have a chance to bind to the natural receptors found on the surface of the cells. In doing so, they render TNF biologically inactive. This helps to reduce joint inflammation associated with arthritis. It also improves the skin lesions seen in psoriatic arthritis.

DOSAGE AND REGIMEN IN ADULTS

For its first five years on the market, Enbrel® therapy required a twice-weekly injection every three to four days. The total recommended adult dosage was 25 mg twice weekly.

In late 2003, the FDA approved a once-weekly dosage of 50 mg of Enbrel® by injection. The approval was based on clinical studies showing that a 50 mg dosage once a week had a sufficient half-life to sustain the treatment benefit. The once-weekly injection schedule provides the same level of effectiveness with greater convenience for patients or care-givers. Patients have a choice as to how they receive the 50 mg per week. The can either inject twice on the same day using a 25 mg dosage for each injection. Or, they can inject every 72 to 96 hours, which equals two injections every seven days.

DOSAGE AND REGIMEN IN CHILDREN

The recommended dosage for juvenile chronic arthritis (JCA) patients ages 4 to 17 is 0.4 mg/kg of body weight, up to a maximum of 25 mg per dose. The drug is injected twice weekly. The child may also be prescribed additional medications to be taken during Enbrel® therapy. These include glucocorticoids, NSAIDs, and some other analgesics. Simultaneous use of methotrexate and Enbrel® has not been studied in pediatric patients, and therefore, its safety has not been established in children with JCA.

CONTRAINDICATIONS

Enbrel® therapy is contraindicated in people with a known allergy to the drug or any of its components, as well as in pregnant or nursing women. The drug should not be prescribed to people who are predisposed to infection. This includes patients with advanced or poorly controlled diabetes, or for those with a history of recurring infections. Tuberculosis has been diagnosed in a small percentage of patients taking Enbrel®, therefore all patients should undergo a tuberculin skin test prior to beginning Enbrel® therapy.

Full prescribing information is available in the product insert sheet. Your doctor may be able to provide you with this insert, or you can download the information from the manufacturer's website at www.amgen.com, or www.enbrel.com.

CLINICAL STUDY FINDINGS

Numerous clinical trials have demonstrated the effectiveness of Enbrel® in adults with RA, psoriatic arthritis, ankylosing spondylitis and juvenile chronic arthritis. Study data on a number of these key trials are summarized in Appendix A.

SAFETY PROFILE IN ADULTS

In clinical studies, a large majority of patients who tried Enbrel® responded to therapy. Most tolerated the drug well, with only 4 percent of participants choosing to discontinue therapy due to side effects. Like all TNF blockers, Enbrel® can cause side effects that range from bothersome to life-threatening or fatal. A discussion of potential risks associated with all TNF blockers is provided in Chapter 5. Following are specific side effects and precautions as they relate exclusively to the clinical experience with Enbrel®.

Most Common Side Effects

The most common side effects were injection site reactions (ISRs), infection and headache. ISRs and infection are described in detail below.

Autoantibody Development

Enbrel® may cause autoimmune antibodies to develop. Clinical studies have shown that a higher percentage of patients taking Enbrel® alone developed new positive anti-nuclear antibodies[32] (ANA) than patients on placebo (11 percent versus 5 percent).

Another study[33] that directly compared ANA in patients taking Enbrel® alone versus those taking methotrexate alone found that the rate of autoantibody development was comparable among both patient groups.

Blood Disorders

There is a slight risk of developing an abnormal blood condition while taking Enbrel®, which can increase your risk of

32 Anti-nuclear antibodies (ANA) are a marker for certain autoimmune conditions such as lupus.

33 Bathon JM, Martin RW, Fleischmann RM, et al. A comparison of etanercept and methotrexate in patients with early rheumatoid arthritis. *N Engl J Med.* 2000;343:1586-1593.

developing a life-threatening infection. In post-marketing[34] experience, several patients taking Enbrel® developed leukopenia (low white blood cell counts), pancytopenia (a reduction in all types of blood cells), or aplastic anemia (a decrease in bone marrow functioning that results in lower red blood cell counts). Some of these patients subsequently died.

Although a definitive link between the blood disorder and Enbrel® has not been established, neither has it been ruled out. It is important to note, too, that most patients on Enbrel® have also taken many other types of arthritis drugs that are also potentially implicated in certain blood disorders. Regardless, if you have a fever or any sign or symptom of infection (e.g., fever, cough, etc.), bruising, bleeding or paleness, you should discontinue Enbrel® and notify your physician immediately.

Cancer (Malignancy)

Lymphomas have been observed in patients taking TNF blockers. In clinical trials, patients taking TNF antagonists showed a higher incidence of lymphoma than the rate expected among the normal adult population as calculated from the National Cancer Institute's SEER database. (SEER is a program of the National Cancer Institute that provides information about cancer incidence and survival in the United States.) It is generally accepted that people with severe, active RA have a greater risk of developing such lymphomas. So it is unknown if the higher incidence of lymphomas among patients on TNF

---

34 Post-marketing is a term used by the FDA to describe events that occur after the drug is approved for commercial marketing.

blockers can be attributed to use of these drugs, or if it is due to the natural course of RA.

Central Nervous System Disorders

There have been a few post-marketing reports of people developing multiple sclerosis (MS) or having a worsening of pre-existing MS while taking Enbrel®. Although there have been no studies to definitely confirm or disprove a connection between MS and Enbrel®, the medical literature supports a possible connection between MS and all TNF blockers. If you have been diagnosed with MS or have a history of optic neuritis or another demyelinating disorder, your physician will probably exercise caution before prescribing a TNF blocker such as Enbrel®.

Congestive Heart Failure

Two large clinical trials that evaluated the effect of Enbrel® in congestive heart failure (CHF) were terminated early due to lack of benefit. Results were mixed. In one study, there was a higher rate of death among Enbrel® patients, although the analysis did not identify specific factors related to CHF. Results from the second study did not corroborate the findings of the first trial. However, there have been post-marketing reports of worsening of CHF in patients taking Enbrel®. There have also been rare reports of newly diagnosed CHF in Enbrel® patients with no known pre-existing heart disease. Until more data are available, physicians should exercise caution when prescribing Enbrel® in patients with heart failure, and the drug should be avoided in patients with moderate to severe heart failure (NYHA class III or IV; see page 91 for an explanation of CHF classes). Heart failure patients taking Enbrel® should be monitored regularly by a cardiologist.

Fertility, Pregnancy and Nursing

The effect of Enbrel® on fertility, pregnancy, and in nursing mothers/infants has not been studied in clinical trials, and no conclusions may be drawn regarding its safety in these situations. Because of the potential adverse effects on the developing fetus or a nursing infant, you should always consult with your physician if you plan to become pregnant, suspect you are pregnant, or intend to nurse your infant while taking Enbrel®.

Infections

In controlled trials, there were no differences in infection rates among patients with RA, psoriatic arthritis, or ankylosing spondylitis. The most common type of infection was upper respiratory infection, which occurred in about one-fifth of both Enbrel® and placebo-treated patients.

With regard to serious infection, clinical studies have shown that the rate of infection is about equal among both Enbrel® patients and patients taking placebo. There have also been post-marketing reports of patients developing serious, life-threatening infections during Enbrel® therapy. Some of these serious infections, including tuberculosis[35], resulted in death.

---

35 American College of Rheumatology *Hotline*. FDA advisory committee reviews safety of TNF inhibitors. September 2001.

For this reason, Enbrel® therapy may be contraindicated in people predisposed to infection, such as is the case with uncontrolled diabetes, congestive heart failure, kidney failure or an immunosuppressive disease. You must never start on Enbrel® therapy during an active infection, and you should inform your physician if any sign of infection occurs.

> 66 I had to stop therapy for three months last year because of the cost, and I thought I would die. After returning to Enbrel®, I felt better in one week. 99
>
> — Sharon Rogers, 48, began Enbrel®
> for RA in January 1999

Injection Site Reactions

The most common adverse effect to Enbrel® in adult clinical studies was injection site reaction (ISR). Nearly 2 of every 5 patients had ISRs, which were described as mild to moderate redness, with or without itching, pain or swelling, at the site of the injection. The average duration of the reaction was three to five days, and some patients experienced a reaction at a previous injection site when a subsequent injection was given. ISR was the only adverse effect that occurred in a higher percentage of Enbrel® patients than in patients injecting placebo.

Your doctor can prescribe a topical steroid cream to help with symptoms. Make sure you notify your physician if the area is not improving to ensure that a skin infection has not developed.

SAFETY PROFILE IN CHILDREN

Juvenile chronic arthritis patients (ages 4 to 17) who participated in the Enbrel® trial generally had the same type of common adverse effects as adult clinical trial patients.

Infection occurred among 62 percent of the participants during Enbrel® therapy. These infections were generally mild and similar to infections commonly seen among normal pediatric populations. Some side effects occurred more frequently in the pediatric participants, as compared with adult study participants. These included headache, abdominal pain, nausea and vomiting.

There were several serious adverse reactions among pediatric clinical study patients taking Enbrel®. These included varicella infection, inflammation of the digestive tract, depression, skin ulcer, blood infection, diabetes mellitus, and soft-tissue and post-operative wound infection. To minimize the possibility of varicella infection (chicken pox), it is recommended that JCA patients comply with all immunization guidelines before starting on Enbrel®.

The long-term safety of Enbrel® has not yet been established in children. Nor has the medication been studied in children younger than 4 years of age.

USE OF OTHER MEDICATIONS WHILE TAKING ENBREL®

Specific drug interactions have not been studied in conjunction with Enbrel® use in adults. Some RA medications can be continued safely during Enbrel® therapy. For adults, these include methotrexate, glucocorticoids, salicylates, NSAIDs, or other analgesics, as prescribed by your doctor. Enbrel® should not be used with other biologic DMARDs (e.g., Kineret®, Remicade® and Humira™).

There is limited experience with the use of Enbrel® and other drugs. No data are available regarding how patients taking Enbrel® respond to a vaccination or a secondary transmission of vaccination by live virus, although vaccines with live viruses (such as those for smallpox and yellow fever) are not recommended. Intranasal live virus flu vaccines, such as FluMist™, should also be avoided.

There is limited clinical experience regarding the use of Enbrel® with other non-RA-specific drugs. Consult your physician or pharmacist if you have questions about specific medications.

SUMMARY: KEY DIFFERENCES BETWEEN ENBREL® AND OTHER TNF BLOCKERS

ENBREL®	REMICADE®/HUMIRA™
FDA approved for early-stage and moderate to severe RA	FDA approved for moderate to severe RA only
FDA approved for RA, psoriatic arthritis, ankylosing spondylitis and JCA	FDA approved for RA only
Injected twice weekly	Injected weekly or twice monthly (Humira™) Infused bimonthly (Remicade®)

IS ENBREL® RIGHT FOR YOU?

Chapter 9 will help you to evaluate if Enbrel® is an option for you. But you may also have a choice of two other

TNF blockers — Remicade® and Humira™. Chapters 7 and 8 review these two drugs in more detail.

CHAPTER 7

Remicade® (Infliximab)

Julie Ewing was eager to try an intravenous (IV) TNF blocker. With a job that required up to six days a week on the road, the requirements of refrigeration and self-injection had their downside. Plus, after a year on an injectable TNF blocker, she seemed to be getting less relief, even with the addition of methotrexate and prednisone.

Julie's decision to try Remicade® couldn't have been better timed. Two months after starting the IV therapy, the 43-year-old was transferred across the country to head up the first phase of a $4 billion project for her employer. Remicade® has helped her to keep up with the demands of the job, which include standing for long periods of time. She still takes methotrexate and prednisone, but the swelling in her left knee is gone, and the flare-ups in her right knee are infrequent and controllable.

Not only is Julie able to handle the long days on her feet, but she is swimming three days a week and feels like she might soon be swinging a golf club again — if she can squeeze in a tee time between weekend hiking trips, and cooking for friends. Now seven months into Remicade® therapy, Julie says this is the closest she has felt to being her "old self" since she was diagnosed with RA five years ago.

REMICADE®: THE ONLY TNF ANTAGONIST AVAILABLE AS AN IV

Remicade® was introduced in the United States in November 1999. It is approved for adults with moderate to severe RA who have not responded to methotrexate alone. Like all TNF blockers, it is used to decrease the number of painful and swollen joints in RA, as well as slow the progression of disease. Remicade's generic name is infliximab (pronounced in-flix-eh-mab).

IMPORTANT FACTS ABOUT REMICADE®

A key difference between Remicade® and Enbrel® or Humira™ is that Remicade® was approved by the FDA based on its positive results in combination with methotrexate. The addition of methotrexate maximizes treatment benefit while minimizing the risk of infusion reactions. (Infusion reactions are described in more detail on page 117.)

Remicade® is also approved to treat Crohn's disease. Crohn's disease is an inflammatory disease of the digestive tract.

An important consideration in Remicade® therapy is that the drug has a long half-life. This means that it stays in your body for a relatively long time. While this can be beneficial in sustaining the drug's effect, it may also pose an increased risk of complications from infection, because the drug can not be eliminated quickly from your system. Staying aware of your general health and calling your physician at the first sign of infection is an important part of Remicade® treatment.

REMICADE® AT A GLANCE

Generic name	Infliximab
Introduced	1999
Manufacturer	Centocor, Inc.
Approved uses	Moderate to severe RA
Delivery	IV infusion
Frequency	Every 4-8 weeks after start-up therapy*
Dosage	3 mg/kg of body weight (max. 10 mg/kg)
Annual cost	$11,766-$62,512**

* The starting regimen consists of an infusion at weeks 0, 2 and 6, then every 8 weeks thereafter.

** Cost varies according to the dosage and frequency of infusions.

HOW REMICADE® WORKS

Remicade® is a recombinant, chimeric[36] IgG1 monoclonal antibody specific for the human tumor necrosis factor. When Remicade® is infused into the body, it floods the system with Remicade® molecules, which bind specifically to TNF-α and block its interaction with the p55 and p75 TNF receptors on the cell surface. This effectively neutralizes the effect of the excess TNF-α molecules found in the synovial fluid in joints, as well as the bloodstream. Excess TNF is implicated in both the pathologic inflammation and the joint destruction that are the primary features of rheumatoid arthritis. (Refer to Chapter 5 for details about TNF and the science behind TNF blockers.) Remicade® and Humira™ work in a similar fashion to bring

---

36 Chimeric refers to the diverse composition of the active component of Remicade®, which is derived from a combination of human and mouse proteins.

relief from an overactive immune response, which is implicated in both rheumatoid arthritis and Crohn's disease.

DOSAGE AND REGIMEN

Remicade® is administered by intravenous (IV) infusion. The IV must be administered by a healthcare professional in a clinical setting. This setting may be a physician's office, an outpatient clinic, or a hospital. The infusion takes about two to three hours. The usual starting dosage is 3 mg per kilogram (kg)[37] of body weight.

When you start on Remicade®, you will undergo three infusions during the first six weeks of therapy. The initial infusion (week 0), is followed by infusions at weeks 2 and 6. Once this initial regimen is completed, you will need to have an infusion only once every eight weeks. It averages out to about six treatments per year.

Patients who experience an incomplete response to Remicade® therapy may be considered for an increased dosage to 10 mg/kg per infusion, or a more frequent dosing schedule of every four weeks.

COMBINATION REMICADE®/MTX THERAPY

Remicade® is typically given in combination with a stable dosage of methotrexate (MTX). This combined therapy maximizes treatment benefits and minimizes side effects. The dosage of methotrexate used in clinical studies ranged from

---

37 A kilogram equals 2.2 pounds. Thus, a 150-pound person weighs about 68 kg.

10 mg to 25 mg weekly. The effectiveness of Remicade®/MTX combination therapy with lower dosages of methotrexate has not been studied.

> 66 Since I have had RA for 47 years, it's hard to remember what life was like before. But the treatment has been everything I hoped for. I rarely have any pain, and I've been able to travel extensively and resume my love of dancing. 99
>
> — Marissa Wentworth, 71, began Remicade® for RA in September 2000

CONTRAINDICATIONS

Remicade® therapy is contraindicated in people with a known allergy to the drug or any of its components, as well as in pregnant or nursing women. The drug should not be prescribed to people who are predisposed to infection. This includes patients with uncontrolled diabetes, or those with a history of recurring infections. Tuberculosis has been diagnosed in a small percentage of patients taking Remicade®. Therefore all patients should undergo a tuberculin skin test prior to beginning Remicade® therapy.

The therapy should be avoided in patients with moderate to severe congestive heart failure (New York Heart Association Class III/IV). If Remicade® is prescribed to a patient with congestive heart failure, the maximum treatment dosage should not exceed 5 mg/kg of body weight.

Full prescribing information is available in the Remicade® product insert sheet. Ask your doctor for a copy of this insert, or you can download the information from the manufacturer's website at www.centocor.com or www.remicade.com.

CLINICAL STUDY FINDINGS

Several clinical trials have demonstrated the safety and effectiveness of Remicade® in adults with RA. Study data from key trials are summarized in Appendix A.

> **66** Allow a half day for treatments. It may seem like a lot of trouble, but the benefits outweigh any inconvenience the treatments may cause. **99**
>
> — Hannah Pembroke, 87, began Remicade®
> for RA in September 2001

SAFETY PROFILE

Remicade® was generally well tolerated by patients in clinical trials, but as with all TNF antagonists, there is a risk of adverse effects. These include the development of serious infections and other illnesses. In some cases, these illnesses resulted in death. A discussion of potential risks associated with all TNF blockers is provided in Chapter 5. Specific side effects and precautions as they relate exclusively to the clinical experience with Remicade® follow here.

Most Common Side Effects

The most common side effects seen with Remicade® include upper respiratory infections, headache, nausea, cough and diar-

rhea. These were considered mild by most clinical study participants. Fewer than 1 percent of patients taking Remicade®
withdrew from treatment due to bothersome side effects.

Autoantibody Development

Remicade® therapy may result in the formation of
autoantibodies. These antibodies sometimes develop into a
lupus-like condition that usually presents as a rash or
another type of arthritis. In clinical studies, more than half[38]
of Remicade® users who tested negative for anti-nuclear antibodies[39] (ANA) at the start of treatment tested positive for
ANA during their treatment. This compared with 19 percent
of patients on placebo. Even so, reports of lupus or lupus-
like symptoms are rare.

"Neutralizing" antibodies that seemed to decrease the
effectiveness of Remicade® developed in a small group of
patients. The addition of methotrexate led to reduced antibody formation and better treatment outcomes.

Cancer (Malignancy)

An increase in the incidence of cancer and lymphomas has
been observed in clinical study participants taking TNF blockers. However, the incidence of malignancies was similar to
what would be expected in the general population. It is generally known that people with severe, highly active RA have a

---

38 This compares to ANA development in 15 percent of Enbrel® users and 12
   percent of Humira™ users.

39 Anti-nuclear antibodies are a marker for certain autoimmune conditions such
   as lupus.

higher risk of developing such lymphomas, so it is not clear whether the cases of lymphoma were due to the therapy or the disease process.

Central Nervous System Disorders

TNF-blocking agents, including Remicade®, have been associated with rare cases of development of a demyelinating disorder (such as multiple sclerosis) or worsening of a pre-existing condition. Remicade® should be used with caution in patients with pre-existing or newly diagnosed central nervous system demyelinating disorders.

Congestive Heart Failure

In clinical trials that evaluated the effect of Remicade® on congestive heart failure (CHF), there was an increased incidence of hospitalization or death due to worsening heart failure in patients receiving more than 10 mg/kg of body weight. Data from more recent clinical trials have produced mixed results with regard to the influence of TNF blockers on CHF. Until more definitive data are available, all other treatment options should be considered in CHF patients before proceeding with Remicade®, and Remicade® should not be used in people with moderate to severe CHF. (Some cardiologists recommend against the use of TNF blockers in anyone with CHF.[40]) If Remicade® is used in a patient with CHF, the maxi-

---

40 Weaver, AL (Chairperson). The evolution of the treatment paradigm of rheumatoid arthritis: cytokine-mediated disease and current therapies. *REACH Continuing Medical Education Monograph.* Released October 2003. Available through Amgen Inc.

mum dosage should not exceed 5 mg/kg of body weight. The patient should also be monitored regularly by a cardiologist.

Infusion Reaction and Infusion Site Reactions

Remicade® may cause an infusion reaction in some patients. Symptoms include, but are not limited to: itching, stinging and chills; and nausea, fever, facial flushing, headache or low blood pressure. In rare instances, life-threatening allergic reactions have been reported.

Patients may also notice an infusion site reaction, which is described as redness, swelling and/or itching at the infusion site. Such reactions nearly always occurred during initial treatments and usually lessen in severity as treatment progresses.

Pregnancy and Nursing

Remicade® should not be used by women of child-bearing age who are not using reliable birth control, because the risk of birth defects is not known. Remicade® has not been studied in women who are breastfeeding, and is not recommended for use by nursing mothers. While taking Remicade®, you should always consult with your physician if you plan to become pregnant, suspect you are pregnant, or intend to nurse your infant.

Additionally, if you are sexually active and taking combination Remicade®/methotrexate therapy, you should use reliable birth control. This precaution applies to both women and men because methotrexate is known to cause birth defects.

Tuberculosis

A rare but potential side effect of TNF antagonist therapy is tuberculosis infection.[41] Tuberculosis was diagnosed in a very small percentage of patients who have taken TNF blockers.

A review of clinical data that included combined statistics for Enbrel® and Remicade® users found more cases of tuberculosis diagnosed with Remicade® (82 of 270,000 patients) compared with Enbrel® (11 of 270,000 patients). This translates to a combined infection rate of less than 0.0003 percent More than three-quarters of these cases of tuberculosis involved patients living outside of North America. Those most at risk for tuberculosis infection while taking TNF inhibitors include people who have lived in endemic regions (for example, certain regions of Europe), as well as patients who take prednisone regularly.

Other risk factors for developing tuberculosis or another opportunistic infection include IV drug users, as well as patients with diabetes, chronic kidney failure, lymphoma, silicosis, or HIV-positive status. Recent immigrants from areas of the world with high rates of tuberculosis or other opportunistic infections are also at higher risk for developing infections while undergoing treatment with a TNF blocker. All patients considering Remicade® — or any other TNF blocker — are advised to undergo a tuberculin skin test prior to beginning treatment.

---

41 American College of Rheumatology *Hotline.* FDA advisory committee reviews safety of TNF inhibitors. September 2001.

Other Infections

As with all TNF blockers, there have been a few reports of serious infections resulting in death among patients taking Remicade®. Therefore, you should tell your physician if you have a history of chronic infections or a condition that puts you at increased risk for complications from infection, such as uncontrolled diabetes.

While on Remicade® therapy, you should also report any sign or symptom of infection (such as fever, cough or skin redness) to your physician immediately. He or she will decide if you should discontinue Remicade® or begin on antibiotic therapy.

Re-Treatment With Remicade®

Discontinuation of Remicade® followed by re-treatment at a later time has resulted in allergic reactions in some people, some of which were serious. Reactions included, but were not limited to, rash, elevated liver function, fatigue and fever.

USE OF OTHER MEDICATIONS WHILE TAKING REMICADE®

Some RA medications — in addition to methotrexate — can be continued safely during Remicade® therapy. These include glucocorticoids, salicylates, NSAIDs or other analgesics, as prescribed by your doctor. Remicade® should not be used with other biologic DMARDs.

There is limited experience with the use of Remicade® and other drugs. No data are available regarding how patients tak-

ing Remicade® respond to a vaccination or a secondary transmission of vaccination by live virus, although vaccines with
live viruses should be avoided. These include vaccines for
smallpox and yellow fever, as well as intranasal spray vaccines
such as FluMist™. Talk with your physician or pharmacist if
you have questions or concerns.

SUMMARY: KEY DIFFERENCES BETWEEN REMICADE® AND OTHER TNF BLOCKERS

REMICADE®	ENBREL®/HUMIRA™
FDA approved for moderate to severe RA	FDA approved for early-stage and moderate to severe RA (Enbrel®) FDA approved for moderate to severe RA (Humira™)
FDA approved for Crohn's disease	—
Stopping/restarting treatment may cause allergic reaction	—
IV infusion	Subcutaneous injection
Infused every 4-8 weeks	Injected twice weekly (Enbrel®) or every 1-2 weeks (Humira™)
Administered at a clinic/doctor's office	Administered at home
Covered by Medicare and most other insurers	Not currently covered by Medicare, but covered by most other insurers

DO YOU PREFER REMICADE® AS A TNF BLOCKER?

So how does Remicade® stack up against Enbrel®? Is it the
right TNF blocker for your situation? Before you decide, read on
about Humira™, the third option in anti-TNF therapy.

CHAPTER 8

Humira™ (Adalimumab)

For Leah Connolly, Humira™ offered the chance to discontinue methotrexate — a drug that provided relief but not without the worry of side effects. Leah, a cytotechnologist, had been on Enbrel® therapy since June 2000. She had gotten good results, but only with the addition of methotrexate.[42] The combination therapy had worked wonders. It relieved the inflammation, pain and stiffness in her fingers, hands and wrists, and her knees were totally pain free. She was once again able to pick up her needlepoint projects and work as long as she wished. At work, she could sit long days at the microscope, handling slides and making fine control adjustments.

But still, the risks of long-term methotrexate use nagged at her. Under Dr. Zashin's care, she weaned herself off the methotrexate and discontinued Enbrel® before starting on Humira™. The 51-year-old lost ground at first, but with every dose of Humira™, she feels better and better. She likes the convenience of Humira™, too. The pre-filled syringes eliminate the

---

42 Not all patients require the addition of methotrexate to TNF antagonist
   therapy to receive benefit from the treatment.

need to mix and prepare the medication, and she only has to inject herself twice a month rather than twice a week.

HUMIRA™: YET ANOTHER GOOD OPTION IN ANTI-TNF THERAPY

Humira™ (pronounced hue-meer-ah) was introduced in the United States in December 2002. The newest of the TNF antagonists, it is approved for adults with moderate to severe RA who have not responded to other DMARDs. In clinical studies, Humira™ was shown to decrease the number of painful and swollen joints in RA, and slow the progression of the disease. Humira's generic name is adalimumab (pronounced a-da-lim-u-mab).

IMPORTANT FACTS ABOUT HUMIRA™

Humira™ is supplied in pre-filled syringes that need to be refrigerated at 36°F to 46°F (2°C to 8°C). Like the other TNF blockers, patients have reported significant improvement within four weeks of the first injection, but it can take up to three months to see a positive response.

HOW HUMIRA™ WORKS

Humira™ is a recombinant, fully human IgG1 monoclonal antibody specific for the human tumor necrosis factor. Humira™ works much like Remicade® to generate its beneficial anti-inflammatory effect in adults with rheumatoid arthritis. The drug, once injected, floods the system with Humira™ molecules, which bind specifically to TNF-α and block its interaction with the p55 and p75 TNF receptors on the cell surface. This effectively neutralizes the effect of the excess TNF-α molecules found in the synovial fluid of the joints as well as the bloodstream. Excess TNF is implicated in both the pathologic inflammation and the joint destruction that are the primary features of rheumatoid arthritis. (Refer to Chapter 5 to learn more about TNF and the science behind TNF blockers.)

HUMIRA™ AT A GLANCE

Generic name	Adalimumab
Introduced	2002
Manufacturer	Abbott Laboratories
Approved uses	Moderate to severe RA
Delivery	Subcutaneous injection
Frequency	Every 1-2 weeks
Dosage	40 mg
Annual cost	$16,488-$32,976*

* Cost varies according to the frequency of injections.

DOSAGE AND REGIMEN

Humira™ is administered by subcutaneous injection once every 14 days. The usual dosage is 40 mg.

If you have a partial response and are not taking methotrexate, your physician may recommend that you inject weekly instead of every other week. This more-frequent dosing regimen has been approved by the FDA. Humira™ should not be taken by people who are allergic to the drug or any of its components. These components include sodium phosphate, sodium citrate, citric acid, mannitol and polysorbate 80. The needle cover on the pre-filled syringe contains dry natural rubber, which may cause an allergic reaction in people with a sensitivity to rubber or latex.

CONTRAINDICATIONS

Humira™ therapy is contraindicated in people with a known allergy to the drug or any of its components, as well as in pregnant or nursing women. The drug should not be prescribed to people who have an active infection, or who are predisposed to infection. This includes patients with uncontrolled diabetes, or those with a history of recurring infections. Tuberculosis has been diagnosed in a small percentage of patients taking TNF blockers. All patients should undergo a tuberculin skin test prior to beginning Humira™ therapy.

Full prescribing information is available in the Humira™ product insert sheet. Your doctor may be able to provide you with this insert, or you can download the information from the manufacturer's website at www.abbott.com, or www.humira.com.

CLINICAL STUDY FINDINGS

Several clinical trials have demonstrated the safety and effectiveness of Humira™ in adults with RA. Refer to Appendix A for details of these studies.

SAFETY PROFILE

Humira™ was generally well tolerated by patients in clinical trials, but as with all TNF antagonists, there is a risk of adverse effects. These include the development of serious infections and other illnesses. In some cases, these illnesses resulted in death. A discussion of potential risks associated with all TNF blockers is provided in Chapter 5. Specific side effects and precautions as they relate exclusively to the clinical experience with Humira™ follow here.

Most Common Side Effects

The most common side effect with Humira™ therapy was a mild injection site reaction (ISR). ISRs were experienced by 20 percent of patients injecting Humira™. ISRs are manifested by a rash, redness, swelling, itching or bruising at the injection site.

Fewer than 10 percent of patients discontinued Humira™ therapy due to adverse side effects. Among these patients, the most common reasons for discontinuing the therapy was an allergic reaction (0.7 percent), rash (0.3 percent) and pneumonia (0.3 percent).

Autoantibody Development

In clinical trials, 12 percent[43] of patients treated with Humira™ developed autoantibodies that are clinical markers for lupus or a lupus-like syndrome. This compared to 7 percent of patients taking placebo. However, only 1 of more than 2,330 patients actually developed lupus. This patient improved once Humira™ treatment was discontinued.

Like Remicade®, a small group of patients taking Humira™ developed "neutralizing" antibodies that seemed to decrease the effectiveness of Humira™. The addition of

---

43 This compares to ANA development of up to 62 percent of patients taking Remicade® and 15 percent of patients taking Enbrel®.

methotrexate led to reduced antibody formation and better treatment outcomes.

Cancer (Malignancy)

An increase in the incidence of cancer and lymphomas was observed in patients taking Humira™ over a period of 24 months in clinical trials. However, the incidence of malignancies was similar to what would be expected in the general population. It is generally known that people with severe, highly active RA have a higher risk of developing such lymphomas, so it is not clear whether the cases of lymphoma were due to the therapy or the disease process.

Central Nervous System Disorders

TNF-blocking agents, including Humira™, have been associated with rare cases of development of a demyelinating disorder (such as multiple sclerosis) or a worsening of pre-existing demyelinating condition. Humira™ should be used with caution in patients with pre-existing or newly diagnosed central nervous system demyelinating disorders.

Congestive Heart Failure

Humira™ has not been specifically studied in congestive heart failure (CHF), and clinical studies of the influence of TNF blockers on CHF have produced mixed results. Until more data are available, caution should be used before prescribing Humira™ in patients with CHF, and the drug should be avoided in patients with moderate to severe heart failure (NYHA class III/IV; see page 91 for an explanation of CHF classes). When

Humira™ is prescribed for patients with heart failure, close monitoring by a cardiologist is recommended.

Fertility, Pregnancy and Nursing

Humira™ has not been studied in pregnancy or in women who are breastfeeding, so its effect on the fetus, the mother and the nursing infant is not known. You should always consult with your physician immediately if you plan to become pregnant, suspect you are pregnant, or intend to nurse your infant while taking Humira™.

> 66 My pain is much less, but I am still limited because of the damage to my joints before starting anti-TNF therapy. My advice to other RA patients is to start it as soon as possible! 99
>
> — Angie Pruett, 35, started Humira™ therapy as part of a clinical trial in June 2000

Infections

As is the case with all TNF blockers, there have been a few reports of serious infections resulting in death among patients taking Humira™. These infections included tuberculosis and infections caused by bacteria or fungi (sepsis).

To minimize your risk of infection, a tuberculin skin test is recommended, and you should not begin Humira™ therapy if you have an active infection of any kind. Your physician will also proceed with caution if you have a history of chronic infections, or if you have a condition that puts you at increased risk for complications from infection, such as uncontrolled diabetes.

During Humira™ treatment, it is important to report any sign or symptom of infection (such as fever, cough or skin redness) to your physician immediately.

USE OF OTHER DRUGS WHILE TAKING HUMIRA™

Certain RA medications can be continued while taking Humira™. These include methotrexate, glucocorticoids, salicylates, NSAIDs or other analgesics, as prescribed by your doctor. Humira™ should not be taken with other biologic DMARDs.

There are limited data regarding the use of Humira™ with other non-RA-specific drugs. No data are available regarding how patients taking Humira™ respond to a vaccination or a secondary transmission of vaccination by live virus. However, vaccines with live viruses are not recommended. These include vaccines for smallpox and yellow fever, as well as intranasal vaccines such as FluMist™.

Although Humira™ has been used in combination with certain RA drugs, specific drug-to-drug interaction studies have not been conducted to date. If you have questions about specific drug interactions, ask your physician or pharmacist.

SUMMARY: KEY DIFFERENCES BETWEEN HUMIRA™ AND OTHER TNF BLOCKERS

HUMIRA™	REMICADE®/ENBREL®
Injected twice monthly	Injected twice weekly (Enbrel®) or Infused every 4-8 weeks (Remicade®)
Supplied to patient in pre-filled syringes	Patient must mix medicine prior to injection (Enbrel®)

IS HUMIRA™ YOUR BEST OPTION?

Now that you have reviewed the TNF blockers as a category and as individual therapies, you can begin to make an informed choice about whether anti-TNF therapy is an option for you, and which is the best drug for your situation. Chapters 9 and 10 will help you sort out the pros and cons of both the therapy and the drugs.

CHAPTER 9

Is Anti-TNF Therapy an Option for You?

Anti-TNF drugs work. The experience of thousands of patients shows that about 2 of every 3 adults who try the therapy respond with at least a 20-percent improvement in their symptoms.

Most patients report less pain and swelling, less morning stiffness, and greater levels of energy throughout the day. By all accounts, Enbrel®, Remicade® and Humira™ offer new hope for an improved health-related quality of life.

But how do you know if the therapy is right for you?

The decision matrix on the following page is a good place to start. For each question that you answer "yes," give yourself the indicated number of points. Tally up your points and compare your total score with the listed recommendations. Then talk with your doctor about what you've learned — together you can decide if this breakthrough therapy is an option for you.

THE TNF BLOCKER DECISION MATRIX (FOR ADULTS WITH RA)

	YES	NO	YOUR SCORE
1. Were you diagnosed with RA within the last 0-24 months?	+2	0	
2. Were you diagnosed with RA within the last 2-5 years?	+1	0	
3. Does your morning stiffness last 45 minutes or more?	+1	0	
4. Do you have 3-6 swollen and tender joints?	+1	0	
5. Do you have 7-12 swollen and tender joints?	+2	0	
6. Do you have 13 or more swollen and tender joints?	+3	0	
7. Have you tested positive for the rheumatoid factor (RF)?	+1	0	
8. Have you tested positive for anti-cyclic citrullinated peptide (CCP) antibodies?	+2	0	
9. Is your erythrocyte sedimentation rate (ESR) elevated?	+1	0	
10. Is your C-reactive protein (CRP) elevated?	+1	0	
11. Do your x-rays show joint damage?	+2	0	
12. Have you tried any of the following medications without success: Ridaura® (auranofin), Plaquenil® (hydroxychloroquine sulfate), Minocin® (minocycline hydrochloride) or Azulfidine® (sulfasalazine)?	+1	0	
13. Have you tried any of the following medications without success: methotrexate (i.e., Rheumatrex®), Arava® (leflunomide), Imuran® (azathioprine), injectable gold (i.e., Myochrysine®), or Cuprimine® or Depen® (penicillamine)?	+2	0	
14. Are you willing to learn to give yourself injections?	+1	0	

Your Total Score [ ]

Interpreting Your Score

12+ points. You are an excellent candidate for TNF blocker therapy, and should ask your physician to prescribe it for 90 days to see if you respond.

However, your physician may proceed with caution, or recommend against TNF antagonist therapy if you have any one or more contraindications to the therapy. These include, but are not limited to, an active infection or another condition that could increase the risk of infection, insulin-dependent diabetes, severe kidney or liver disease, moderate to severe congestive heart failure (NYHA class III/IV), multiple sclerosis, open wounds or a history of recurring infections.

9-12 points. You may be a good candidate for TNF blocker therapy, and should ask your physician about prescribing it for you. Of course, if you have a contraindication to TNF antagonist therapy, as described above, your physician may postpone or recommend against it.

5-8 points. TNF blocker therapy may still be an option for you, but there may be other, better alternatives for your RA. Your physician can help you decide on the best therapy for your condition and medical history.

4 or fewer points. TNF blocker therapy is probably not an option for your condition. Your physician is your best resource to help you explore and decide on an appropriate treatment for your RA.

10

CHAPTER 10
—
Choosing the Right TNF Blocker

Enbrel®, Remicade® and Humira™ are all effective in treating certain types of arthritis, and rheumatoid arthritis (RA) specifically. As explained in Chapter 5, these biologic DMARDs target overproduction of tumor necrosis factor (TNF). TNF is one of the biological processes that causes pain, inflammation and joint damage in rheumatoid arthritis and related conditions such as psoriatic arthritis and ankylosing spondylitis. In clinical studies, all three anti-TNF drugs were found to be similar in their effectiveness in treating the signs and symptoms of rheumatoid arthritis, as well as in slowing the progression of the disease. They also have similar safety profiles.

So if you and your doctor have determined that anti-TNF therapy is an option for you (refer to Chapter 9), how do you know which of the three drugs is best for your specific situation?

The answer lies in understanding the four key differences between these three drugs, and how they relate to your condition, lifestyle and personal preferences.

THE FOUR KEYS TO SELECTING A TNF BLOCKER

While many factors may influence the decision about which TNF antagonist is best for you, the decision comes down to four key factors.

1. RA, JCA, Ankylosing Spondylitis or Psoriatic Arthritis

Enbrel®, Remicade® and Humira™ are all FDA-approved to treat rheumatoid arthritis. However, only Enbrel® is also FDA-approved for psoriatic arthritis, ankylosing spondylitis, and juvenile chronic arthritis.

2. Methotrexate or Not

The FDA recommends that Remicade® be used only in combination with methotrexate. So if you opt for Remicade® therapy, it is recommended that you also take methotrexate. Many patients do not require the addition of methotrexate to achieve significant benefit with anti-TNF therapy, and taking methotrexate is optional with Enbrel® and Humira™. In addition, other DMARDs may be used optionally with all three TNF blockers.

3. Injection Versus Infusion

Enbrel® and Humira™ are given by injection at home. You can inject the drug yourself, or a caregiver can administer the injections. Enbrel® requires two injections per week, either twice on the same day or once every 72 to 96 hours. Enbrel® must first be prepared by mixing the drug with a liquid. Humira™ requires one injection every one to two weeks. Humira™ is supplied in a pre-filled syringe.

Remicade® requires an intravenous (IV) infusion, which must be performed in a clinical setting, such as an outpatient clinic, a hospital infusion center or your physician's office. After an initial start-up period, Remicade® infusions are typically administered once every eight weeks. The infusions generally take about two to three hours.

4. Cost

TNF antagonists are costly, ranging from about $12,000 to more than $60,000 per year depending upon which drug you are prescribed and your dosing frequency. Many major health insurers provide pharmacy benefits for these drugs. An exception is Medicare, which covers only Remicade® therapy. (As of the date of publication, Medicare doesn't cover self-injectable drugs, so Enbrel® and Humira™ are not covered.) If cost is an issue — and it is for most people — be sure to review your health insurance plan to determine what benefits may be available to help with the cost of TNF blocker therapy.

For patients with health insurance. If TNF antagonists are covered by your insurance plan, you will need to follow your insurer's guidelines about what authorizations are needed, how to fill prescriptions, what you will have to pay up front or as a co-payment, how you will be reimbursed for the expense of your first dosage, and if you must file a claim. (Some of these details may or may not be applicable to your situation.)

Your physician's billing office may be able to help you determine what pharmacy benefits are available to you and how best to fill your prescription or schedule an appointment with an infusion clinic.

Another good source of help is through the drug manufacturers (see page 152). All three have patient support programs to help you make the transition to TNF antagonist therapy. Their services generally include assistance in determining your health insurance pharmacy benefits.

With your written permission, a manufacturer-sponsored reimbursement professional will contact your insurance company to determine if your insurance policy covers the therapy, what specific benefits are available, and what prescription parameters are required. If your plan does not require that you use a specific or contracted pharmacy supplier, the manufacturer's patient support representative can also help you to locate either a mail-order pharmacy or a pharmacy close to your home. The manufacturers also have experience in handling claim denials, and may be able to provide some suggestions if your insurance company denies coverage for anti-TNF therapy.

Be prepared to provide the manufacturer's patient support representative with the following information:

- Your name, address, date of birth and Social Security number
- The name, address and phone number of your insurance company
- The name, address, date of birth and Social Security number of the policyholder (if other than you)
- The policyholder's employer, the employer's address and phone number, and the policy or group number
- A daytime phone number where you can be reached

You will also be required to sign and return a written release that allows your physician to share information about your medical history with the manufacturer to the extent required to help determine availability of benefits.

For patients with Medicare. Medicare currently does not provide a prescription drug benefit, so Enbrel® and Humira™ are not covered benefits for most Medicare patients. (Some secondary insurance plans cover these drugs, however, so be sure to check with your secondary insurer if you have one.) Remicade®, because it is an infusion therapy administered in a clinic, is presently a covered Medicare benefit.

If you are a Medicare patient and prefer the idea of an injectable TNF antagonist but have no pharmacy benefits to defray the costs, you may still have another option. Humira's manufacturer (Abbott Laboratories) has a Medicare assistance program that provides the drug at no charge to eligible Medicare patients. You can apply for the program through your physician. There are no guarantees that you will qualify, but you still may want to give it a try if you are a Medicare patient interested in an injectable TNF blocker.

For uninsured or underinsured patients. If you do not have health insurance, or if your insurance plan offers no or inadequate pharmacy benefits, you may still have access to anti-TNF therapy. Most pharmaceutical companies have patient assistance programs that temporarily provide prescription drugs at no cost to eligible patients based on financial need. All of the manufacturers of TNF blockers have such programs in place. Your physician and/or his staff can provide additional information on whether you might qualify and how you can apply for these programs (also see page 152).

THE DECISION IS YOURS

Since Enbrel®, Remicade® and Humira™ are essentially equivalent in terms of safety and effectiveness, which drug is best for you is really a matter of your diagnosis and personal preference.

If you have psoriatic arthritis or ankylosing spondylitis (or if you have a child with JCA), the "best" TNF antagonist for your situation is fairly straightforward. Only Enbrel® is currently FDA approved for these rheumatic conditions. Even so, some physicians may opt to prescribe another of the TNF antagonists for psoriatic arthritis or ankylosing spondylitis. This is a fairly common practice called "off-label" use. (Remicade® and Humira™ are currently being studied for these applications.)

If you have rheumatoid arthritis, you have three good choices: Enbrel®, Remicade® or Humira™. Your physician can offer guidance, but truly, the best TNF blocker for your situation is the one that you prefer, can tolerate and can afford.

To help you make the choice, ask yourself: Do I prefer an injection or an IV infusion? Do I want to inject twice a week or twice a month? Am I willing to learn how to self-inject? Would my partner or caregiver be willing to inject me? Is it more convenient to go to a clinic once every eight weeks for a two- to three-hour infusion? Do I want to try to control my arthritis with one medication or is a combination therapy better? What does my health insurance cover?

The following chart may help you to sort out these issues. (A comprehensive comparison of Enbrel®, Remicade® and Humira™ begins on page 143.)

FACTORS THAT MAY INFLUENCE YOUR CHOICE OF TNF BLOCKER

		ENBREL® (Etanercept)	REMICADE® (Infliximab)	HUMIRA™ (Adalimumab)
Diagnosis	RA – adult/early-stage	✓		
	RA – adult	✓	✓	✓
	RA – juvenile (JCA)	✓		
	Psoriatic arthritis	✓		
	Ankylosing spondylitis	✓		
Lifestyle/personal preferences	Prefer injections over IV infusions	✓		✓
	Prefer IV infusions over injections		✓	
	Fewest number of treatments		✓ (6-12x/yr)	
	Fewest number of injections			✓ (2-4x/mo)
	Prefer treatment at home	✓		✓
	Prefer treatment at the doctor's office or a clinic		✓	
	Are not willing to learn to self-inject		✓	
	Do not want to mix medication		✓	✓
	Prefer one arthritis medication to a combination	✓		✓
	Cannot tolerate methotrexate	✓		✓
Insurance	Insurance with pharmacy benefits	✓*	✓*	✓*
	Medicare only		✓	✓**
	Medicare plus a secondary insurer	✓*	✓*	✓*
	No health insurance or underinsured	***	***	***

* Benefits vary. Always check with your insurer before committing to therapy.

** Through the manufacturer's Medicare Assistance Program.

*** Eligible uninsured and/or underinsured patients may qualify for the manufacturer's Patient Assistance Program, which can be applied for only through the prescribing physician.

If you have a preference for one drug over another, make your preferences known. If only one TNF blocker is being recommended to you, ask your doctor if one of the other TNF blockers might be a better alternative. The important thing is that both you and your physician keep an open line of communication in matters related to your health care and your treatment options.

> 66 There are always some negative things said about side effects, but I discuss them with my doctor until I am comfortable. 99
>
> — Connie Garrett, 71, began TNF blocker therapy for RA in June 2003

If you get no response from the first TNF blocker you are prescribed within 90 to 180 days, ask to be prescribed one of the other TNF blockers. If this drug fails to provide relief, it is not unreasonable to ask your physician to prescribe the third TNF blocker, or consider adding methotrexate. As long as you are willing and in generally good health, there is no reason not to try to get the life-changing benefits of TNF antagonist therapy.

COMPARING THE TNF BLOCKERS

	ENBREL® (Etanercept)	REMICADE® (Infliximab)	HUMIRA™ (Adalimumab)
Description	TNF antagonist	TNF antagonist	TNF antagonist
U.S. introduction	November 1998	November 1999	December 2002
Composition	100% human fusion protein	75% human protein; 25% murine (mouse) protein	100% human TNF monoclonal antibody
FDA-approved uses	• Early-stage RA • Moderate to severe RA • Psoriatic arthritis • Ankylosing spondylitis • Polyarticular juvenile chronic arthritis	• Moderate to severe RA • Crohn's disease	• Moderate to severe RA
Contraindications	• Allergic to the drug or any of its components • Active infection • Open wound • History of recurring infections • Active tuberculosis • Congestive heart failure • Severe kidney or liver disease • History of lymphoma • Multiple sclerosis	• Allergic to the drug or any of its components • Active infection • Open wound • History of recurring infections • Active tuberculosis • Congestive heart failure • Severe kidney or liver disease • History of lymphoma • Multiple sclerosis	• Allergic to the drug or any of its components • Active infection • Open wound • History of recurring infections • Active tuberculosis • Congestive heart failure • Severe kidney or liver disease • History of lymphoma • Multiple sclerosis

COMPARING THE TNF BLOCKERS (continued)

	ENBREL® (Etanercept)	REMICADE® (Infliximab)	HUMIRA™ (Adalimumab)
Storage	• Refrigerate at 36°F to 46°F (2° to 8°C) • Keep out of direct light	Not applicable — not dispensed to patients	• Refrigerate at 36°F to 46°F (2° to 8°C) • Keep out of direct light
Administration	• Requires mixing of drug with sterile water and filling syringe • Subcutaneous injection • Injection given by patient or caregiver at home	• Packaged in a ready-to-use IV bag with tubing • Intravenous infusion • Administered at a clinic or physician's office	• Packaged in a ready-to-use syringe • Subcutaneous injection • Injection given by patient or caregiver at home
Dosage frequency	Once per week via 2 injections on the same day — OR — Twice per week (every 72-96 hours)	6-12 times per year, as follows: 2-hr infusion at week 0, week 2, and week 6; then every 4-8 weeks thereafter	Once every 2 weeks — OR — Once every 1 week if not taking MTX
Maximum dosage	25 mg per injection; 50 mg total per week	3-10 mg/kg of body weight per infusion	40 mg every 1-2 weeks
Used with methotrexate?	Optional	Yes; MTX ≥ 10 mg daily	Optional

	ENBREL® (Etanercept)	**REMICADE®** (Infliximab)	**HUMIRA™** (Adalimumab)
Used with DMARDs other than MTX?	Optional (although not studied)	Optional (although not studied)	Optional (although not studied)
Side effects — common*	• Injection site reaction • Upper respiratory infection	• Infusion site reaction • Infusion reaction • Upper respiratory infection • Headache • Nausea • Fatigue	• Injection site reaction • Upper respiratory infection
Side effects — infrequent*	• Headache • Nausea • Dizziness • Cough • Rash • Chest pain • Back pain	• Urinary tract infection • Dyspepsia (stomach symptoms) • Fever • Hypertension • Back pain • Abdominal pain • Dizziness • Cough • Diarrhea	• Headache • Nausea • Dizziness • Cough • Fever

* Other side effects may have been reported that are not listed here.

COMPARING THE TNF BLOCKERS (continued)

	ENBREL® (Etanercept)	REMICADE® (Infliximab)	HUMIRA™ (Adalimumab)
Side effects — rare*	• Sepsis (serious infection) • Tuberculosis • Multiple sclerosis and other demyelinating disorders • Heart failure • Liver failure • Kidney failure • Aplastic anemia • Drug-induced lupus • Lymphoma • Blood disorders	• Sepsis (serious infection) • Tuberculosis • Multiple sclerosis and other demyelinating disorders • Heart failure • Liver failure • Kidney failure • Drug-induced lupus • Lymphoma	• Sepsis (serious infection) • Tuberculosis • Multiple sclerosis and other demyelinating disorders • Heart failure • Liver failure • Kidney failure • Drug-induced lupus • Lymphoma
Approx. annual retail cost	$16,488 (52 weeks at 50 mg per week)	$11,766-$62,532 (52 weeks at 2-7 vials every 4-8 weeks, including infusion fees)	$16,488-$32,976 (52 weeks at 40 mg every 1-2 weeks)
Covered by health insurers?	Yes, by most; but always verify benefits with your insurer	Yes, by most; but always verify benefits with your insurer	Yes, by most; but always verify benefits with your insurer
Covered by Medicare?	No**	Yes	No**; but the manufacturer offers a Medicare assistance program

* Other side effects may have been reported that are not listed here.

** As of publication date

TAKING THE NEXT STEP: TALKING WITH YOUR PHYSICIAN

Here are some important issues to discuss with your doctor before you begin treatment with a TNF antagonist.

Combination Therapy With Methotrexate

In adults, Enbrel® and Humira™ therapy is approved for use with or without methotrexate. Combining a TNF blocker with methotrexate often increases its benefit. (Methotrexate is generally always used in combination with Remicade® therapy.) If you are currently taking methotrexate, ask your physician if you will continue taking methotrexate once you start on Enbrel® or Humira™. If you will continue methotrexate, more frequent monitoring via laboratory tests is recommended. In up to one-third of patients, the methotrexate dose may be able to be decreased and eventually discontinued.

The Use of Other RA Drugs

Certain RA medications have been used safely in combination with TNF blockers. These include glucocorticoids, salicylates, NSAIDs, other analgesics, or methotrexate (described above). Ask your physician if the combination of a TNF blocker with other medications requires any special precautions.

Possible Unwanted Side Effects

TNF blockers are generally well tolerated, but like all drugs, they can cause adverse side effects. For the injectable TNF blockers, the most common side effect is injection site reactions. Up to 37 percent of patients taking Enbrel® and 8 percent of those taking Humira™ experience injection site reactions. You should also note that the plastic needle cover on the syringe used to inject these drugs is lined with latex. This can cause a reaction if you have an allergy to latex. Be sure to talk to your doctor about alternatives.

Upper respiratory infections are another common ailment among people taking TNF blockers. Other side effects occurred much less frequently, including headache and nausea. There were also some cases of serious infections that resulted in death. Your physician can explain more about side effects of each of these drugs to you in detail. Or, you can learn more by downloading prescribing information from the manufacturer's websites at www.enbrel.com, www.remicade.com, and www.humira.com.

Injections

Enbrel® requires two injections every week. Humira™ requires an injection every one to two weeks. A nurse, pharmacist, or other healthcare professional can teach you or a caregiver how to prepare the injection and administer the shots at home. Be sure to talk with your physician about how and when this training will take place.

It is a good idea to receive your first injection in your physician's office. This ensures that the medication is injected properly and allows the staff to monitor you for an adverse reaction.

If at First You Don't Succeed…

Lack of success with one TNF blocker does not necessarily exclude success with the others, as these patients can attest:

- Victoria Archer got instantaneous relief from Humira™, after 12 weeks on Enbrel® offered no benefit at all. Angie Pruett received no benefit from Humira™, but Enbrel® has improved her mobility to the point where she is traveling again.

- Benjamin Banks was prescribed Remicade® during a temporary Enbrel® shortage in 2002. Remicade® improved his psoriatic symptoms by more than 90 percent during 10 weeks on the therapy. He started Enbrel® in 2003. It has maintained his "new, clear skin," while also improving his joint symptoms by another 10 percent.

- Carla Mason had several years of success on Enbrel®, but discontinued it for financial reasons when her COBRA insurance coverage expired. Remicade® proved ineffective, and Carla felt fortunate to qualify for Humira's patient assistance program. Still, when she was again eligible for employer-sponsored health insurance, Carla restarted on Enbrel®, which has given her excellent results with few side effects.

- Sarah Olson has also been on all three TNF blockers. Enbrel® provided initial good results but the relief diminished after a year. She switched to Remicade®, but had an adverse reaction. Sarah started on Humira™ plus methotrexate about a year ago, and is again getting good results with the recent addition of Arava®. Sarah concedes that her RA has been difficult to treat, but she never loses hope. "Since the addition of Arava®, I have been completely free of RA symptoms and have had no side effects. I am an artist, enjoy golf and hiking. Anti-TNF therapy has allowed me to again participate in the things I love."

Infusion

Remicade® requires an IV infusion that must be administered by a licensed healthcare professional in a clinic or
physician's office. Be sure to talk with your physician about
where you will go for the infusion therapy. Many physicians
offer this service at their offices or an affiliated outpatient
center.

Ask if Benadryl® (diphenhydramine hydrochloride)
and/or Tylenol® (acetaminophen) will also be given during
therapy. These drugs are sometimes given to help minimize
side effects. Benadryl® can cause drowsiness, so you may want
to have someone drive you home after infusion treatment if
Benadryl® will be part of your therapy.

> 66 You can adjust to any inconvenience when you feel as well as
> I do. 99
>
> — Rose Gordon, 61, began TNF blocker
> therapy for RA in October 2001

Immunizations

Data regarding the safety and effect of vaccinations during
TNF antagonist therapy are limited. The current thinking is
that live vaccines (e.g., vaccines for smallpox and yellow fever)
should not be administered to patients taking TNF blockers.
Inactivated or killed vaccines, such as those for flu or pneumonia, are felt to be safe. Be sure to ask for your physician's
guidance before getting any kind of vaccine.

Insurance Coverage

As mentioned earlier, TNF antagonists are expensive. The cost may preclude anti-TNF therapy as a treatment option for people who are uninsured or underinsured. Your physician and his staff will likely have had a good deal of experience in dealing with this situation, so don't be embarrassed to ask for advice and assistance.

Even for patients who have adequate insurance coverage for anti-TNF therapy, additional or ongoing approvals may be required by the health insurance plan. This is why it is critical that you understand your insurance benefits before you start treatment. Ask your physician or call the manufacturer for help in determining what benefits are available to you under your health plan, and how you can maximize those benefits to minimize your out-of-pocket costs. If the insurance company declines to cover the cost of the medication, ask your physician if he or she will write a letter on your behalf. This document, called a "letter of medical necessity," should describe your condition and medical history, including previously failed treatment and the potential benefits of TNF blockers. It should be written to present a strong case to support reimbursement for TNF-blocking therapy for your specific situation.

If you have no pharmacy benefits, ask your physician for help in determining if you qualify for a manufacturer-sponsored patient assistance program. And if you are a Medicare patient who would like to try Humira™, but have no pharmacy benefits available to you, ask your physician to contact the manufacturer to see if you qualify for its Medicare assistance program.

HELP IS JUST A PHONE CALL AWAY

	ENBREL® (Etanercept)	REMICADE® (Infliximab)	HUMIRA™ (Adalimumab)
Manufacturer	Amgen Inc.	Centocor, Inc.	Abbott Laboratories
Patient support program	Enliven®	RemiCARE™	InteRAct™
Toll-free number	(888) 4-ENBREL (888) 436-2735	(866) REMICARE (866) 736-4227	(800) 4-HUMIRA (800) 448-6472
Web address	www.enbrel.com	www.remicade.com	www.humira.com
Insurance questions	(888) 4-ENBREL (888) 436-2735	(800) 964-8345	(800) 4-HUMIRA (800) 448-6472
Special programs for uninsured or underinsured patients	• Patient assistance program	• Patient assistance program	• Patient assistance program • Medicare assistance program

After you talk to your physician, are cleared for a TNF antagonist, and know how you will cover the cost of the therapy, you'll be eager to get started. Chapter 11 describes what to expect during this potentially life-changing therapy.

Getting Started on a TNF Blocker

Getting started on TNF blocker therapy requires a team effort between you and your healthcare provider. You'll be taking a new and proactive role in your arthritis treatment. To be successful, you will need to show a willingness and ability to perform new tasks, including managing an injection or infusion schedule. Many people feel overwhelmed by the process at first. But the anxiety tends to quickly fade as comfort and confidence are gained — especially when you begin to feel well again.

MAKING THE COMMITMENT

Any new drug regimen requires a commitment of time and energy, as well as a willingness to learn a new program and stick to it. Patience is important, too. Some people respond to TNF-blocking therapy within the first two weeks, but it may take longer — three months or more — for you to see benefit.

The medication is administered by regularly scheduled injections (Enbrel® and Humira™) or intravenous infusions

(Remicade®). Most patients learn to self-inject either on their own or with the help of a friend or family member. This allows them to manage their therapy at home.

The commitment to Remicade® may be easier for some people to manage because it is administered as an IV infusion at a clinic or doctor's office. Still, it is important to maintain a regular infusion schedule and to keep your infusion appointments.

If anti-TNF treatment is well tolerated and no serious side effects occur, the TNF blocker will likely become a permanent part of your life — a long-term therapy requiring long-term compliance.

FILLING YOUR PRESCRIPTIONS

Filling and refilling prescriptions is an issue only with Enbrel® and Humira™. (Remicade® is administered in a clinic, so you will not have to worry ordering the medicine.)

Allowing adequate lead time for prescription refills is a must. Because of the cost and special handling requirements, some mail-order plans and local pharmacies do not keep a supply on hand for immediate pick-up or shipment. It is important to contact your pharmacist or plan administrator about how much lead time is required to order and obtain Enbrel® or Humira™.

Fill times of three to five days are typical for local pharmacies. Many mail-order plans require at least two weeks, plus the time required to ship the medication to you — so you may have to order your prescription three weeks or more before you will need it. Remember, too, that regardless of whether you pick up your prescription or have it delivered, it will need to be refrigerated at 36°F to 46°F (2°C to 8°C) as soon as you receive it. Enbrel® and Humira™ should never be frozen. Nor should they be left in direct sunlight or outdoors in a hot or cold environment for an extended period of time.

GETTING TO KNOW THE TOOLS OF YOUR THERAPY — ENBREL®

Your pharmacy provides Enbrel® to you in a carton. Each carton contains four dose trays, which represents a two-week supply. The "dose tray" is actually a cardboard box, which holds the items you will need to prepare and inject the medication:

- 1 vial, containing 25 mg of Enbrel® powder
- 1 syringe, pre-filled with a liquid (called a "diluent") that is mixed with the Enbrel® powder
- 1 vial adapter, which is used when reconstituting a single dose
- 1 27-gauge, 1/2-inch long needle
- 1 plunger, which is used in conjunction with the syringe
- 2 alcohol swabs, which are used to cleanse the injection site before and after the injection
- 4 "mixing date" stickers to indicate when you mixed the Enbrel® powder with the diluent

The carton, the Enbrel® vial and the syringe label are stamped with the expiration date. Make it a habit to look at this date before you prepare Enbrel® for dosing. All expiration dates should be the current month and year or later. If any component of the dose tray is out of date, do not use it. Call your physician or pharmacist for instructions.

GETTING TO KNOW THE TOOLS OF YOUR THERAPY — HUMIRA™

Humira™ is supplied as a pre-filled, ready-to-use syringe in a dose tray. The tray also includes an alcohol prep pad and an instruction card with a drawing of the pre-filled syringe. The package and pre-filled syringe are marked with the expiration date. Make it a habit to look at this date before you inject. All expiration dates should be the current month and year or later. If the package is out of date, call your physician or pharmacist for instructions.

LEARNING TO LIVE WITH INJECTIONS

For many patients, the biggest hurdle of injectable TNF blocker therapy is learning to accept weekly or biweekly shots for an indefinite period of time.

You are in good company if you have a fear of needles or a reluctance to self-inject. But every successful patient will also tell you that the benefit of the injection far outweighs the fear of a needle stick. In fact, some patients actually look forward to the injection because of the relief it brings.

Your physician's medical staff will teach you to self-inject. Some patients already have experience with injections; for example, those who self-inject methotrexate for RA, or insulin for diabetes. Thus, they need only minimal guidance to get started on TNF blocker therapy.

The majority of patients have no experience in giving injections, and so the learning curve is steeper. Regardless, the thousands of patients around the world who are successful Enbrel® and Humira™ users should be evidence enough that you, too, can learn to self-inject.

---

66 One day I just closed my eyes and pushed the needle. After that it was easy. **99**

— Peter Stewart, 31, began injectable TNF blocker
therapy for RA in December 2002

Before you begin your treatment, ask your physician or nurse for any patient information provided by the manufacturer. Or, contact the manufacturer yourself. All three manufacturers have patient support programs that provide useful information, helpful services and ongoing product updates to patients and medical professionals. For Enbrel® users, Amgen Inc. offers a resource kit that includes a video tape, a handbook, and some other tools that you may find helpful. Special travel coolers are also available to patients through the patient support program, which is called the Enliven® program. Patient programs are also available for Humira™ (the InteRAct™ program) and Remicade® (the RemiCARE™ program). Refer to page 152 for phone numbers and Internet addresses of these manufacturers.

For the first injection — and probably until you are comfortable with injecting yourself — you will go to your physician's office to watch, listen, ask questions and practice. You will have to bring the medication, syringe, etc. Your physician provides only the prescription for Enbrel® or Humira™, but not the drug itself.

> 66 Sign up for the manufacturer's patient support services. They augment the instructions from the doctor's office. 99
>
> — Theresa Cunningham, 59, began TNF blocker therapy for RA in November 2002

In the controlled setting of your physician's office or clinic, you will learn about sterile technique, preparing the medication properly, handling a syringe, administering a subcutaneous (under the skin) injection, caring for the injection site, and safely disposing of the syringe and needles. The medical staff will be able to monitor you for any signs of serious or life-threatening allergy during your initial treatment.

Don't expect to learn everything during the first session. It takes most people two or more one-on-one sessions until they are confident, comfortable and competent in handling the injection on their own.

MAKING INJECTABLE TNF BLOCKERS PART OF YOUR ROUTINE

Enbrel® and Humira™ are unlike any other medications on the market. Understanding their special handling requirements will make it easier to work this new drug regimen into your routine — and move you one step closer to successful treatment.

Because these drugs are human proteins that are manufactured using DNA technology, they must be refrigerated to preserve the proteins. The safe temperature range is 36°F to 46°F (2°C to 8°C).

Before you can inject Enbrel®, the white refrigerated powder must first be reconstituted. This requires mixing the powder with a liquid called a diluent. The diluent activates the Enbrel®. Reconstituting the powder is a delicate process that takes about five to 10 minutes.

It is best to inject Enbrel® as soon as possible after it has been reconstituted. However, in a pinch, you can re-refrigerate the reconstituted Enbrel® at 36°F to 46°F (2°C to 8°C) for up to 14 days. Enbrel® should never be frozen in either its powder or reconstituted form.

During your early experience with Enbrel®, the treatment may take you 30 minutes or more to perform. This is normal. As you become more experienced with using Enbrel®, you may be able to complete your treatment in 15 minutes or so.

Humira™ is supplied in pre-filled syringes for added convenience.

The important thing is that you allow yourself enough time to safely and comfortably perform the treatment. Select a time when you are clear-minded and unhurried. Perhaps you will choose to get up earlier on treatment days, when your household is quiet and you have sufficient time to concentrate on the task. Or perhaps your best time for injection is before you go to bed, when you are relaxed and winding down.

Enbrel® is injected twice weekly (either twice on the same day; or one injection every 72 to 96 hours, which works out to about twice a week). Humira™ is injected once every one to two weeks. It doesn't matter whether you inject in the morning, afternoon or evening. What is important is that you inject on a consistent schedule throughout treatment, administering the medicine at regularly scheduled intervals. Many people find that maintaining a calendar is the best way to stay on track with your dosing schedule.

MAINTAINING A POSITIVE OUTLOOK

It may take some time to notice a benefit from TNF blocker therapy. A small number of patients have reported feeling better after their first injection or infusion. More than likely, it will take two, four, or even 12 weeks before you begin to respond. So patience and perseverance are absolutely essential to success with this therapy.

Remember, too, that not everyone who tries TNF blocker therapy benefits from it. Up to 1 of every 3 patients does not respond optimally to the treatment. And still other patients have adverse reactions that cause them to discontinue the treatment. So while you should remain vigilant about possible adverse side effects, keep a positive outlook, too. It will help to improve your mood and lift your spirits during the initial weeks of the therapy.

KNOWING WHEN TO ASK FOR HELP

TNF antagonist therapy is an entirely new experience that will take time to learn. Feeling slightly overwhelmed by numer-

Traveling Tips for Injectable TNF Blockers

"Traveling is a bit of a hassle, but not a problem," says Annie Pearson, 66, an experienced traveler when it comes to flying with an injectable TNF blocker. Planning ahead minimizes inconveniences:

1. Ask your physician for a general letter that states your diagnosis and explains that you manage your condition with self-injected medication. You'll rarely need the letter, but it will speed you through a security checkpoint if a question arises.

2. Always pack your meds in your carry-on bag. Make sure your medication is properly labeled (with the manufacturer's and/or pharmacy's label) and has not expired. Notify the security screener if you are carrying a sharps container in your carry-on bag.

3. Keep the medication cool using a small, insulated lunch bag and freezer packs. The freezer packs last 6 to 8 hours on a warm day. Pamela Williams, who has been traveling with an injectable TNF blocker since 2003, packs plastic zippered freezer bags, too. The bags can be refilled with ice twice a day and at night to keep the medication cool if your hotel room doesn't have a refrigerator.

4. If you're traveling with kids, Susan Holt offers a simple tip to save space: pack your TNF blocker medication with the baby's bottles.

5. Susan Holt also offers a solution for safely disposing of syringes and needles while staying in a hotel room: a compact disposable sharps container that she orders through her pharmacy. These containers range in size from 0.6 - 1.4 quarts. Among the smallest is the 2" x 2" x 7" Sharp Trap® (made by Harbor Safety). Several manufacturers make small (4" x 4" x 8") transportable containers. Some can be purchased online.

ous details during your first several treatments is perfectly normal. A bit of anxiety is also to be expected when you inject at home or go to the clinic for the first time. But with time and attention, you will grow comfortable with this therapy.

Still, there are times when you need to contact your physician for advice.

If You Have an Infection

The effect of TNF antagonists on the immune system is not well understood. What is known is that their mechanism of action suppresses the immune system, which increases the risk of infection. During clinical trials, minor infections, such as upper respiratory tract infections, were common. There were also several cases of serious infection, and some of these patients died. So it's important to stay aware of your general health. Do not begin anti-TNF therapy if you have an active infection of any kind (either chronic or localized). Contact your physician if you develop a fever, notice redness in a cut or wound, or have any sign or symptom of an infection while taking TNF antagonists. Your physician will decide if you should temporarily discontinue anti-TNF therapy and/or begin antibiotic treatment.

If You Are Scheduled for Surgery

If you are scheduled for surgery, let your doctor know so that he or she can determine the best course of action. Because surgery poses an increased risk of infection, your doctor may want you to discontinue anti-TNF therapy for a week or two weeks before surgery, and resume therapy one week after surgery if you do not develop an infection or another complication.

If a Side Effect Becomes Bothersome

Side effects do occur with TNF blockers, but most are not serious enough to cause patients to discontinue the therapy. However, if any side effect or symptom (e.g., injection site reaction, nausea, vomiting or headache) worsens or becomes bothersome, call your physician and ask for advice.

If You Decide to Discontinue Therapy

If there is not an immediate reason to discontinue therapy, you may want to talk with your doctor before abandoning anti-TNF treatment. TNF-blocking therapy is considered a long-term therapy, and discontinuing treatment may result in the recurrence of your arthritis symptoms. In the case of Remicade®, stopping and restarting therapy has resulted in an allergic reaction in some patients.

If You Are Diagnosed With Diabetes

Diabetes puts you at increased risk for infection, which can make you more susceptible to serious infection while on TNF antagonists. You will need to keep your physician informed if you are diagnosed with diabetes during TNF-blocking therapy.

If You Are Diagnosed With Multiple Sclerosis

There have been post-marketing reports of patients developing multiple sclerosis (MS) or experiencing a worsening of their existing MS during TNF-blocking therapy. No definitive link between TNF blocker treatment and MS has been established, but the medical literature supports this possibility. If you have MS, a history of optic neuritis, or are diagnosed with MS or another demyelinating disorder of the central nervous system, talk with your physician immediately about whether you should continue with TNF-blocking therapy.

If You Plan to Become Pregnant

The effect of TNF antagonists on developing fetuses and nursing infants has not been studied in humans. If you are sexually active, you should use a reliable method of birth control while taking TNF blockers. If you become pregnant, discontinue therapy and notify your physician immediately. If you plan to become pregnant, it is important to discuss your plans with your doctor before discontinuing birth control or TNF-blocking therapy.

Before You Get a Vaccination for the Flu, Pneumonia, Smallpox or Overseas Travel

Vaccines of killed viruses (such as those used to vaccinate against influenza and pneumonia) are considered safe, but there are limited data to confirm this definitively. Vaccines of live viruses (e.g., for smallpox or yellow fever) as well as intranasal live flu vaccines such as FluMist™ are definitely not recommended while on TNF antagonist therapy. The effect of live viruses in people taking TNF blockers has not been studied and may put you at risk for serious infection. Be sure to ask your physician for advice before getting a vaccination of any kind, including shots required for overseas travel. Also talk to your doctor if a member of your household is receiving a live vaccine.

If You Have Any Concerns

If you have questions or concerns about any aspect of your treatment, call your physician.

GETTING MORE INFORMATION

It never hurts to know all you can about a new treatment alternative. More information generally helps you to make a more-rounded and better-grounded decision that fully considers the pros, cons, risks and benefits. It also helps to stay abreast of the latest developments with TNF therapy.

Here are some additional resources that may be able to provide you with information about TNF antagonists, as well as other treatments for arthritis.

Patient Education and Support Organizations

The Arthritis Foundation. P.O. Box 19000, Atlanta, GA 30326. (800) 283-7800. www.arthritis.org.

The National Psoriasis Foundation. 6600 SW 92nd Avenue, Suite 300, Portland, OR 97223. (800) 723-9166. www.psoriasis.org.

Spondylitis Association of America. P.O. Box 5872, Sherman Oaks, CA 91413. (800) 777-8189. www.spondylitis.org.

Professional and Scientific Organizations

American College of Rheumatology. 1800 Century Place, Suite 250, Atlanta, GA 30345. (404) 633-3777. www.rheumatology.org.

National Institute of Arthritis and Musculoskeletal and Skin Diseases (NIAMS), National Institutes of Health. 1 AMS Circle, Bethesda, MD 20892-3675. (301) 495-4484. www.niams.nih.gov.

Pharmaceutical Manufacturers

Abbott Laboratories (maker of Humira™/adalimumab). 100 Abbott Park Road, Abbott Park, Illinois 60064-3500. Humira™ patient line: (800) 448-6472. www.humira.com.

Amgen Inc. (maker of Enbrel®/etanercept). Amgen Center, Thousand Oaks, CA 91320-1799. Enbrel® patient line: (888) 436-2735. www.enbrel.com.

Centocor, Inc. (maker of Remicade®/infliximab). 200 Great Valley Parkway, Malvern, PA 19355. Remicade® patient line: (866) 736-4227. www.remicade.com.

Your Healthcare Team

Your physician and his or her staff are a great source of information about treatment options for arthritis. In addition, they may be able to recommend local patient support groups where you can meet other patients with first-hand experience with TNF blockers.

A FINAL WORD

The decision to undergo TNF-blocking therapy may be one of the biggest commitments you'll ever make. But once you get comfortable with the treatment process and its special requirements, you'll find that it poses little inconvenience in your day-to-day activities. For most people with arthritis, this is the first step in reclaiming a fuller, happier, healthier and more active life.

> 66 My husband gives me the injections. After years of watching me struggle with RA, he feels as if he is able to help me, and knows how much relief the injection brings. 99
>
> — Jill McLeod, 34, began injectable TNF blocker therapy for RA in April 1999

CHAPTER 12

25 FAQs About TNF Blockers

It's always wise to learn all you can about a new treatment before you get underway. That way, you'll know what to expect and when to ask for help. Be sure to take time to carefully review the materials that your physician or nurse gives you about TNF antagonist therapy, and discuss your questions and concerns fully before you begin treatment.

Here are answers to some of the most frequently asked questions (FAQs) about TNF blockers to give you a starting point to dialogue with your healthcare provider. Your physician, nurse or pharmacist can also provide you with additional information as it relates to your specific situation.

1. CAN TNF BLOCKERS CURE MY ARTHRITIS?

No. But they have been shown to slow the progression of structural joint damage (erosion) and joint space narrowing, particularly in early-stage RA. They have also proven effective in reducing the signs and symptoms of arthritis, including painful, swollen and inflamed joints associated with RA and other types of inflammatory arthritis.

2.   WILL TNF BLOCKERS IMPROVE THE APPEARANCE OF MY ENLARGED JOINTS?

Only to the extent that the medication reduces swelling and inflammation, and slows joint erosion. However, TNF blockers do not reverse existing joint deformities.

3.   HOW LONG WILL IT TAKE TO FEEL BETTER?

Some patients say they begin to feel better within 24 to 48 hours of their first injection or infusion. This effect may temporarily taper off during the first days or weeks of therapy, but relief usually returns with continuing treatment. It's important to note that some patients never respond to therapy, but the majority of patients will get benefit within four to six weeks, with maximum benefit attained at 12 weeks.

4.   HOW MUCH BETTER WILL I FEEL?

Patients who responded to TNF-blocking agents in clinical trials achieved at least ACR 20 — a 20-percent improvement in their arthritis symptoms. Many saw improvement to ACR 50 or ACR 70, and limited long-term data show that the benefit appears to be sustained over time. (Refer to the glossary and appendix for a more detailed explanation of ACR 20, 50 and 70.)

5.   IF I FEEL WELL ENOUGH TO EXERCISE, CAN I?

Of course, but use common sense and moderation. Be sure to protect your joints with proper warm-up and cool-down exercises. If you haven't been regularly participating in an exercise program, be sure to get your physician's approval first.

6.   WILL TNF BLOCKER THERAPY ALLOW ME TO STOP TAKING OTHER MEDICATIONS FOR ARTHRITIS AND PAIN?

TNF blockers enable many patients to discontinue or decrease the amount of other medications they take for their arthritis. Depending upon your condition, medical history and current level of pain and inflammation, your physician may choose to continue one or more arthritis medications in addition to the TNF blocker you are taking. If you are prescribed Remicade®, you will usually remain on methotrexate. Methotrexate is optional with Enbrel® and Humira™. TNF blockers have also been used safely with other medications used in arthritis treatment, including glucocorticoids, salicylates, NSAIDs, and some analgesics (e.g., Tylenol® and hydrocodone).

7.   HOW LONG WILL I HAVE TO TAKE A TNF BLOCKER?

TNF blockers are considered a long-term treatment. During clinical trials, patients who stopped taking TNF blockers had a recurrence of their arthritis symptoms within a month. So if you tolerate TNF-blocking therapy without bothersome symptoms or adverse side effects, your physician will probably keep you on the drug indefinitely.

8.   WHAT HAPPENS IF I STOP AND RESTART TNF BLOCKER THERAPY?

If you stop treatment, the drug may provide some lasting relief at first, but most patients find that their arthritis symptoms soon return. If your doctor instructs you to temporarily discontinue the drug (for example, due to an infection), you will probably want to restart it as soon as you can to minimize the return of symptoms. A word of caution, though, about stopping and restarting Remicade®. Discontinuing Remicade® followed by re-treatment with Remicade® has resulted in allergic reactions in some people. (Taking methotrexate may diminish this effect.) If you stop Remicade® for any reason, you may want to consult with your physician before starting back on it.

9.   WILL TNF BLOCKERS MAKE ME SICK?

TNF blockers were well tolerated in clinical trials, but there is always a chance that you will have an adverse reaction. In clinical studies, the most common side effect for injectable TNF blockers was injection site reactions. Upper respiratory tract infections were also common among users of all three TNF antagonists. A small percentage of patients experienced other side effects, including nausea, headache, upset stomach, dizziness or a rash. Contact your physician if you have any side effect that worsens or becomes bothersome, or if you have any sign or symptoms of an infection.

10.   WHAT KIND OF INFECTION IS SERIOUS ENOUGH TO CALL MY DOCTOR?

Because TNF blockers may increase your risk for serious infection, any sign of infection should be reported to your doctor.

Remember, TNF blockers work by removing tumor necrosis factor (TNF) from your body in significant amounts. This is beneficial in treating rheumatic diseases such as RA, psoriatic arthritis and ankylosing spondylitis, but it may also lower your resistance to infection. A small number of patients taking TNF blockers have developed very low white blood counts, which can increase the risk of serious and sometimes life-threatening infections. In clinical studies, some of these infections were fatal. So it is very important that you remain aware of changes in your general health while taking a TNF blocker and notify your physician at the first sign of an infection.

Symptoms and signs of infection include, but are not limited to, sore throat, persistent cough, sinus drainage, cuts that don't heal promptly, or fever. Depending upon your condition, your doctor may order a course of antibiotic treatment, instruct you to temporarily discontinue your TNF blocker, or order additional tests.

11. HOW SERIOUS ARE THE INJECTION OR INFUSION SITE REACTIONS?

In clinical studies, almost half of patients experienced redness, swelling and/or itching at injection or infusion site. Injection or infusion site reactions (ISRs) nearly always occurred during initial treatments, and became less frequent or less severe as treatment continued. The majority of ISRs were mild in nature, and resolved on their own in three to five days. A small percentage of patients also experienced a reaction at previous injection sites when a subsequent dose was injected. Most patients learn to live with ISRs, but you should contact your physician if ISRs persist, worsen, or become bothersome. Applying a topical corticosteroid cream or Benadryl® (diphenhydramine hydrochloride) may also help to reduce the swelling and itching.

12. ARE TNF BLOCKERS SAFE AND EFFECTIVE WHEN USED FOR LONG PERIODS OF TIME?

Compared with medications that have been available for many years, TNF blockers are still relatively new, so there is limited experience with respect to long-term safety and sustained benefit. Based on the data to date, it appears that TNF blockers are able to sustain relief safely in a majority of patients. There is also no indication at this time that the risk of infection increases over the course of treatment. But as with all newer medications, there is a possibility that a new serious adverse effect may present itself in the future as more people take the medication over a longer period of time.

13. ENBREL® HAS BEEN APPROVED BY THE FDA FOR PSORIATIC ARTHRITIS, ANKYLOSING SPONDYLITIS AND JUVENILE CHRONIC ARTHRITIS. ARE REMICADE® AND HUMIRA™ ALSO APPROVED FOR THESE USES?

Not as of the date of this book. However, your physician may prescribe a TNF blocker other than Enbrel® for these conditions, a common practice called "off-label" use.

14. I'M TAKING A TNF BLOCKER NOW, BUT WANT TO START A FAMILY SOMEDAY. WHEN IS IT SAFE TO BEGIN TRYING TO GET PREGNANT?

The effect of TNF blockers on pregnancy and in nursing mothers and infants has not been studied, so safety data are not available. If you are sexually active, you should use a reliable method of birth control while on anti-TNF therapy. If you are thinking about becoming pregnant, suspect you are pregnant, or want to nurse an infant, notify your physician so that you can discuss what is best for you and your baby.

15.   I ALWAYS GET A FLU SHOT. IS THIS A PROBLEM WITH TNF BLOCKERS?

Limited data are available regarding the safety and effectiveness of vaccinations in people taking TNF blockers, so be sure to consult your physician for advice.

A single small study[44] of immune responses to a pneumonia vaccine showed a slightly lowered response among patients taking Enbrel® or Remicade® compared with the control group. This study suggests that inactivated or killed vaccines, such as those for flu, pneumonia, hepatitis A, hepatitis B and toxoid (diphtheria and tetanus), still provide some level of protection against contracting these illnesses. While killed vaccines are felt to be safe, no assurances can be made regarding safety.

Live vaccines, including those given for yellow fever and smallpox (as well as the intranasal flu spray FluMist™), should be avoided if you are taking a TNF blocker. In the case of smallpox vaccines, the U.S. Centers for Disease Control consider anti-TNF therapy to be a contraindication to vaccination, due to the immunosuppressive properties of these drugs.[45]

---

44 Elkayam O, Caspi D, Paran D, et al. Effect of anti-TNF-alpha therapies on the immunogenicity of pneumococcal vaccination in patients with rheumatic diseases. *Arthritis Rheum.* 2002;46(suppl):S861.

45 US Centers for Disease Control. List of medications contraindicating smallpox vaccination receipt. April 25, 2003. Available at http://www.bt.cdc.gov/agent/smallpox/vaccination/immuno_suppress_meds.asp.

Regarding yellow fever vaccination, the CDC cites the theoretical risk of infection for people with compromised immune systems due to either disease (such as HIV infection) or immunosuppressive medications, which includes TNF blockers. Its advisory for international travelers[46] states that such patients should not be vaccinated for yellow fever. If travel to a yellow-fever-infected zone is necessary, the CDC recommends that the patient be advised of the risks posed by such travel, instructed in methods for avoiding mosquito bites, and supplied with vaccination waiver letters by their physicians.

It is also reasonable to avoid contact with people who have recently received a live vaccine, for a limited period of time. Check with your doctor for specific guidelines.

16.   DO TNF BLOCKERS CAUSE UNINTENDED INTERACTIONS WITH OTHER DRUGS?

Specific drug interactions with TNF blockers have not yet been studied, so there is no scientific information about adverse drug interactions. According to *The Medical Letter Handbook of Adverse Drug Interactions*[47], no specific interactions have been recognized to date. Contact your physician if you have questions about any specific drug-to-drug interaction.

---

46 US Centers for Disease Control. Health information for international travel, 2003-2004 (The Yellow Book): yellow fever. June 30, 2003. Available at http://www.cdc.gov/travel/diseases/yellowfever.htm.

47 Kim RB, ed. The Medical Letter Handbook of Adverse Drug Interactions. New Rochelle, NY: The Medical Letter, Inc;2003:525,550.

17.   WHY DO TNF BLOCKERS HAVE TO BE INJECTED OR GIVEN BY IV?

TNF blockers are protein-based medications that are man-ufactured using DNA technology. The active proteins in these drugs are too fragile to withstand digestion. So rather than tak-ing them by an oral route, they are administered by subcutaneous injection or intravenous infusion.

18.   WHAT IF I MISS A INJECTION?

It depends upon which injectable TNF blocker you are tak-ing. Enbrel® injections should not be given more frequently than every 72 hours, so if you miss your shot by more than three days, you should probably wait until your next regular dose. If you are taking Humira™ and miss an injection by a few days, you should probably go ahead and take it as soon as you remember. If you are not sure what to do, call your physician or pharmacist for advice.

19.   CAN I MIX ENBREL® AHEAD OF TIME AND INJECT IT LATER?

It is best to administer Enbrel® immediately after it has been mixed. In an emergency, you can refrigerate the reconsti-tuted dose at 36°F to 46°F (2°C to 8°C). However, the dose must be used within 14 days.

20.   ON SPECIAL OCCASIONS WHEN I WANT TO FEEL MY BEST, I HAVE THOUGHT ABOUT TAKING AN INJECTION AHEAD OF SCHEDULE. WILL THIS HURT ME?

The maximum approved dose of Enbrel® for adults is 50 mg a week. The maximum dosage for Humira™ is 40 mg once weekly.

The effect of higher dosages of these drugs has not been studied. So it is not wise to exceed the maximum recommended dosage. Nor should you increase the frequency of the dose.

21. CAN I MIX THE ENBREL® POWDER WITH TAP WATER?

No. The pre-filled syringe contains a diluent of 1 milliliter of sterile bacteriostatic water, which contains 0.9 percent benzyl alcohol. The diluent supplied in the dose tray is the only liquid that should be used to reconstitute the Enbrel® powder. If you inadvertently spill the pre-filled syringe, set the entire dose tray aside, and use a new one. Then call your pharmacist or physician for instructions.

22. MY PRESCRIPTION DELIVERY WAS DELAYED BY THE SHIPPER BY A DAY. IS IT SAFE TO USE?

Prolonged exposure to heat or extreme cold (below freezing) can spoil Enbrel® or Humira™. Consult your pharmacist or the mail order pharmacy for advice if your prescription arrives at your home in an unrefrigerated (or frozen) condition.

23. WHERE CAN I GET ANOTHER NEEDLE DISPOSAL BOX TO DISPOSE OF MY USED SYRINGES AND NEEDLES?

If there are no children in your household, you can use a clean plastic or cardboard milk carton to hold your used syringes and needles. Be sure to mark the container clearly as medical waste, and dispose of it properly when it is full. If you prefer to use a commercial sharps disposal container, ask your pharmacist about purchasing one.

24.   ARE THE INJECTABLE TNF BLOCKERS MORE EFFECTIVE THAN THE INFUSION TYPE FOR RA?

No. All three medications target the biologic function of TNF, and all three drugs are safe and effective for a majority of patients who use them. Refer to Chapter 10 for a side-by-side comparison of the three drugs.

25.   CAN I TRAVEL WITH ENBREL® OR HUMIRA™?

Absolutely. You'll just need to keep the medication refrigerated at a temperature of 36°F to 46°F (2°C to 8°C) and out of direct light. If you need only to carry one or two dose trays, place the cartons in a thermal lunch bag (or small ice chest) with a freezer/ice pack(s). Some people save the insulated shipping cartons from the mail-order pharmacy just for this purpose. You may also want to contact the drug manufacturer and ask about the availability of a thermal travel case designed specifically for the medicine. Refer to page 152 for contact information.

Refrigerate the dose trays as soon as you arrive at your destination. If you are taking Enbrel®, it is best not to premix your Enbrel® to save space. Pack only complete, prepackaged dose trays, and prepare the dosage following the standard mixing and injection instructions. If your travel plans require more than one or two dose trays, consult with your physician or pharmacist for advice. As with all medications, keep your medication with you. Don't pack it in luggage that will be stowed as checked baggage.

CHAPTER 13

Looking Forward to the Future

In 1979, Demetria Isaacs's future arrived much too quickly. Newly diagnosed with rheumatoid arthritis, the 26-year-old faced daily pain and bouts of self-pity and depression, wondering what her life might have been if not for RA. Now, more than two decades later and four years into TNF blocker therapy, Demetria believes that her best days lie ahead.

"I feel like I've been given my 30s back again. I feel better and it shows in my attitude and my movement. I've joined a health club. I ride an exercise bike, participate in water aerobics, and work out on the machines to build my strength and endurance. After living with pain for more than 20 years, and having tried nearly every treatment for RA with limited success, I never dreamed that I could feel 'normal' again."

TNF blocker therapy has made a believer of Adam Nussbaum, and his family and friends, too. Five years ago, the 60-year-old man's arthritis pain had became the focal point of his life — shutting out his wife, children and friends. Years of medications had ravaged his body, and the pain had engulfed him, body and mind. He was desperate for an answer, and anti-TNF therapy provided it. Today, Adam has reclaimed his life, rebuilt his relationships with his family, and returned to his beloved hobby of building and flying radio-controlled model aircraft.

"My life isn't perfect since I have an illness for which there is no cure. But this therapy has given me back my life and a new appreciation for it. I tell my wife, 'Let's get going. We've got a lot of living to do.'"

Science created TNF blockers and is well on the way to proving that the discovery of such a life-changing treatment was not an isolated event. New biologic treatments for RA are already in the pipeline and showing promise in early clinical research. These include the use of special molecules that prevent bone and joint deterioration, as well as treatments that block interleukins and reduce the level of vascular endothelial growth factor (VEGF), a protein that is involved in the formation of rheumatoid tissue.

A new fusion protein, known as cytotoxic T-lymphocyte-associated antigen 4-IgG1 (CTLA4Ig), is the first of a new class of biologic drugs, much like TNF antagonists, that is currently in development. This new category of drugs is called co-stimulation blockers, and it has produced good outcomes for a majority of RA patients in preliminary clinical studies.

Enbrel® is being studied in other applications, ranging from Alzheimer's disease and ovarian cancer to sciatica. Remicade® and Humira™ are now being studied for application in spondyloarthropathy as well as other non-arthritic conditions. There are also new TNF blockers in development.

All of these exciting research and development initiatives offer ever-increasing treatment options across a broad spectrum of diseases and conditions — and will, perhaps, one day, bring us closer to a cure for rheumatoid diseases like RA.

Still, looking ahead to this future begins with seeing past today's pain. For Adam Nussbaum, Demetria Isaacs, Carla Mason, Julie Barton, Brad Prater, Susan Holt, Leah Connolly, Victoria Archer, Bob Honeywell and tens of thousands of others, discovering TNF-blocking medication has been a miracle — transforming their existence from one of pain to one of movement, and providing them with living proof that life with chronic arthritis can still mean a very bright future: one of active, pain-free living and dreams left to explore.

Key Clinical Studies of TNF Blockers

The body of scientific data regarding TNF blockers is large, growing and ever-changing. This knowledge base dates to the 1990s, when the first TNF antagonists — after showing promise in animal studies — began to be tested in humans. The data generated from these early trials provided the basis for FDA-approval of TNF blockers. These trial data are on file with the FDA. Study data relevant to the individual product approvals (Enbrel®, Remicade® or Humira™) are printed on the package insert that is included with every package or prescription for these products. The data are also available through the manufacturers, and are readily available online. (Refer to page 152 for contact and website information.)

Clinical studies, however, generally continue long after the initial FDA approval. The use of these medications over a longer term is important in validating the long-term safety and efficacy of these medications in the general population.

AN OVERVIEW OF CLINICAL TRIALS

Clinical trials are sponsored or funded by any number of organizations, including pharmaceutical companies, medical foundations, universities and groups of researchers both in the United States and around the world. The U.S. federal government also sponsors clinical trials through agencies such as the National Institutes of Health (NIH), the Department of Defense (DOD), and the Department of Veteran's Affairs (VA). Trials can take place in a variety of locations, including hospitals, universities, doctors' offices and community clinics.

Studying Experimental Drugs

Studies of experimental drugs — medications that have not yet been brought to the marketplace — are conducted in phases. Each subsequent phase has a more specific purpose and generally involves a larger number of participants. For medical products being studied for commercialization in the United States, there are four phases of clinical trials:

Phase I. A Phase I clinical study evaluates the safety, appropriate dosage levels, and general response to a new treatment. The new treatment can be either a pharmaceutical product or a medical device. Because little is known about the possible risks and benefits of the treatment being tested, phase I trials usually include only a small number of patients who have not been helped by other treatments.

Phase II. A Phase II clinical study tests whether a new treatment has benefit in a certain disease process or for a specific medical condition.

Phase III. A Phase III clinical study compares the results of a new treatment against a standard treatment and/or placebo. Based on the safety and effectiveness of the drug as demonstrated in Phase I and II trials, Phase III studies usually involve hundreds or thousands of patients at multiple treatment centers.

Phase IV. A Phase IV clinical study evaluates "post-marketing" side effects in a larger population. Phase IV studies may reveal benefits or adverse reactions that were not apparent in Phase III studies. Phase IV trials take place after a treatment has been approved by the FDA and made available to the general population. Long-term safety data are often the result of manufactured-sponsored, ongoing Phase IV trials.

HOW RESEARCHERS MEASURE IMPROVEMENT IN ARTHRITIS

To understand these results of the clinical studies included in this Appendix, it is also helpful to know how researchers measure "improvement" in arthritis patients. There are generally two measures of improvement: (1) clinical response to the therapy; and (2) health-related quality of life assessments.

Measuring Improvement Through Clinical Response

Patients are first evaluated at the study's outset. This is called the baseline. It provides the "status quo" against which measures of treatment outcomes can be made. Patients are assessed again — either upon attaining a stated clinical objective, and/or at one or more periods ranging from three months to many years. These are called the study's endpoints. A number of tools are used to quantify improvement (or lack thereof) from baseline to endpoint.

ACR Response Criteria System.[48] The American College of Rheumatology (ACR) response criteria system measures clinical response to therapies used to treat RA. The rating indicates the degree of improvement and is expressed as a percentage of improvement.

The ACR rating assesses improvement in three key areas: (1) the number of tender and swollen joints; (2) the patient's and/or physician's subjective assessment of pain, function and disability; and (3) results of certain blood tests called "acute phase reactant tests." These tests, such as erythrocyte sedimentation rate (ESR) and C-reactive protein, measure elevation in certain proteins in the blood in response to inflammation.

Researchers then assess the overall effectiveness of the active drug therapy by comparing it to placebo therapy. (Placebo is a harmless inactive treatment that looks/feels/tastes virtually the same as the real therapy.) Effectiveness of the therapy is gauged by looking at how many patients achieved "ACR 20," "ACR 50," or "ACR 70" at each of the study's end points.

For example, ACR 20 indicates:

• A 20-percent improvement in tender joint and swollen joint count

• Plus, a 20-percent improvement in at least three of the following:

---

48 Felson DT, Anderson JJ, Boers M, et al. American College of Rheumatology preliminary definition of improvement in rheumatoid arthritis. *Arthritis Rheum.* 1995;6:727.

- The patient's assessment of pain
- The patient's global assessment (Overall, how does the patient say she feels?)
- The physician's global assessment (Overall, how does the doctor feel the patient is doing?)
- The patient's assessment of disability (What does the patient say she can and can not do?)

• Plus, a 20-percent improvement in acute phase reactant measures (either ESR or CRP level).

ACR 50 refers to a 50-percent improvement in these three criteria. ACR 70 refers to a 70-percent improvement in these criteria. ACR 70 is the closest clinical measure to remission of RA signs and symptoms.

Disease Activity Score (DAS). The DAS is a clinical tool used to measure the extent of disease activity in RA. The score is calculated by the number of tender and swollen joints in combination with the erythrocyte sedimentation rate.

Total Sharp Score (TSS). The total Sharp score is a method for evaluating changes in total joint damage. It is calculated by assessing the number of bone erosions and the amount of joint space narrowing as seen on x-ray.

Measuring Improvement in Health-Related Quality of Life

Researchers use various measurement systems and tools to objectively report improvements in health-related quality of life. Three of the most frequently used measurement tools are the HAQ, FACIT and SF-36. Because these tools are used by researchers and institutions around the world, they are copyrighted to preserve their validity as a reliable and meaningful measure of clinical outcomes.

Health Assessment Questionnaire (HAQ).[49] The HAQ was originally developed in 1978 by researchers at Stanford University for assessing quality of life among patients with arthritis. The HAQ has also been used to assess health-related quality of life in other medical conditions. The questionnaire depends on patients (rather than a clinician) to self-assess their functional abilities (what they "can do"), and includes measures of disability, pain, overall health, treatment side effects, health resource utilization and demographics. Responses are then scored over time to evaluate differences before, during and after a specific treatment. The HAQ is the most common quality of life measurement tool used in studies of arthritis and arthritis treatments.

Functional Assessment of Chronic Illness Therapy (FACIT).[50] The FACIT measuring system is a collection of questionnaires designed to assess health-related, quality of life issues in people with chronic illnesses. FACIT was first introduced in 1987 with a questionnaire specific for cancer therapy. The questionnaire is divided into four sections: physical well-being, social/family well-being, emotional well-being, and functional well-being. Variations of the cancer-related questionnaire have been used and validated in other chronic illness conditions, including arthritis.

---

49 Bruce B, Fries JF. The Stanford health assessment questionnaire: a review of its history, issues, progress, and documentation. *J Rheumatol.* 2003;30(1):167-178.

50 Webster K, Cella D, Yost K. The functional assessment of chronic illness therapy (FACIT) measurement system: properties, applications, and interpretation. *Health Qual Life Outcomes.* 2003 Dec 16;1(1):79.

Medical Outcomes Study Short Form 36 (SF-36).[51,52] SF-36 is a patient-administered quality-of-life measurement tool that is widely used for non-rheumatologic conditions, but has been studied for application in RA. The tool was designed in a longer format in 1992 for the Medical Outcomes Study. The "36" refers to form's 36 questions that measure general health. SF-36 assesses quality of life in eight areas: physical function; role limitation due to physical health problems; bodily pain; general health perception; vitality; social functioning; role limitations because of emotional health problems; general mental health; and self-reported health transition.

THE LANGUAGE OF CLINICAL TRIALS

Combination therapy. Two or more therapies used concomitantly to treat a condition.

Concomitant. Concurrent; happening at the same time.

Controlled study. A clinical study that includes a comparison group, which is called the control group. The control group may receive a placebo, another treatment, or no treatment at all.

Cross-over. Refers to a clinical study where patients taking placebo are permitted to "cross over" into the experimental treatment group so that they may attempt to get benefit from

---

51 Ware JJ, Sherbourne CD. The MOS 36-item short-form health survey (SF-36). I. Conceptual framework and item selection. *Medical Care.* 1992;30:473-83.

52 Reed PJ. Medical outcomes study short form 36: testing and cross-validating a second-order factorial structure for health system employees. *Health Services Research.* 1998:Dec.

the drug under investigation. Patients receiving the drug under study may also opt to "cross over" to placebo treatment.

Double blind. Refers to a clinical study in which neither the participants nor the researchers know whether the placebo treatment or active treatment is being administered to a given patient. The purpose of double-blind studies is to eliminate bias in evaluating the efficacy of a treatment.

Endpoint. Termination point of a clinical trial, based on the attainment of a clinical status or the passage of a specified period of time.

Extension trial. Extension of a clinical trial beyond its original endpoint.

Efficacy. The effectiveness of a medical treatment.

Monotherapy. A single therapy used to treat a condition.

Multi-center study. A clinical trial that is carried out at more than one site, e.g., multiple clinics or other treatment settings.

Open label. Refers to a clinical trial in which both the participants and researchers know what treatment the participant is taking and at what dose. Open label is the opposite of a blind trial, in which participants and/or researchers do not know what therapy the patient is undergoing.

Placebo. An inactive substance that looks the same and is administered in the same way as a drug in a clinical trial, but has no pharmacologic action against a patient's illness or complaint. In a clinical trial, placebo treatment given to the control group allows the specific and nonspecific effects of the experimental treatment to be measured objectively.

Randomized. Refers to a study in which the participants are assigned randomly to different treatment groups. Random assignment ensures that the treatment groups will be similar, which allows an unbiased evaluation of the treatments.

Single blind. Refers to a clinical study in which researchers know which treatment (including placebo) patients have been assigned to receive, but the patients remain unaware until the end of the trial.

Statistical significance. The use of statistical methods to demonstrate that a result obtained in a clinical trial is due to the treatment being studied, because the probability of obtaining such a result by chance alone is relatively low.

Treatment arm. Treatment group.

THE ARMADA TRIAL

Drug Studied

Humira™ (adalimumab)

Study Title

A̲nti-TNF R̲esearch Study Program of the M̲onoclonal A̲ntibody D̲2E7[53] in Rheumatoid A̲rthritis (ARMADA)

Purpose

The data[54,55] from the ARMADA trial were pivotal in the FDA's decision to approve Humira™. Humira™ is approved for reducing the signs and symptoms of RA, as well as slowing the progression of structural damage in adults with moderately to severely active rheumatoid arthritis (RA) who have had insufficient response to one or more DMARDs.

Trial Design

ARMADA was a 24-week, randomized, double-blind study of 271 patients with active RA despite current treatment with MTX. Patients were randomly assigned to one of four study groups: 20 mg, 40 mg or 80 mg of Humira™ or placebo every other week while continuing to take

---

53 Adalimumab was called D2E7 in earlier phases of product development.

54 Abbott Laboratories news release. Adalimumab improves rheumatoid arthritis disease activity. January 30, 2003.

55 Weinblatt, ME, Keystone EC, Furst DE, et al. Adalimumab, a fully human anti-tumor necrosis factor monoclonal antibody for the treatment of rheumatoid arthritis in patients taking concomitant methotrexate. *Arth Rheum.* 2003;48(1):35-45.

methotrexate. The efficacy of Humira™ was assessed using the American College of Rheumatology ACR 20 response, as well as quality of life measurements using the Health Assessment Questionnaire.

Clinical Results

At 24 weeks, more than half of the patients receiving Humira™ 40 mg every other week achieved an ACR 20 and ACR 50 response (67.2 percent and 55.2 percent). This response was significantly greater than the response achieved in patients receiving placebo (14.5 and 8.1 percent).

Additionally, more than one-fourth of patients achieved ACR 70 (26.9 percent vs. 4.8 percent for placebo). Responses were generally rapid. Some patients reached an ACR 20 response after one week of treatment (25.4 percent of patients receiving Humira™ 40 mg every other week versus 6.5 percent with placebo).

Patients receiving Humira™ plus methotrexate showed a statistically significant improvement at 24 weeks over baseline in each of the seven ACR core components, including tender joint count, swollen joint count, patient pain assessment, and patient global assessment of disease compared to patients receiving methotrexate plus placebo.

Quality of Life Measurements

Quality of life outcomes were measured using the SF-36 questionnaire and the fatigue scale of the FACIT questionnaire. After week 24, improvements in the average SF-36 physical component summary scores and FACIT fatigue scale scores were greater in patients receiving Humira™ 40 mg than those receiving placebo. This improvement was statistically significant.

Adverse Effects

In this study, the most common adverse events seen in patients receiving Humira™ 40 mg compared to placebo were rhinitis (25.4 percent vs. 19.4 percent), upper respiratory tract infection (14.9 percent vs. 9.7 percent), flu syndrome (14.9 percent vs. 8.1 percent), injection site pain (10.4 percent vs. 3.2 percent) and diarrhea (10.4 percent vs. 8.1 percent). Five Humira™ patients withdrew from the study versus 2 placebo patients due to adverse events.

THE ASPIRE TRIAL

Drug Studied

Remicade® (infliximab)

Study Title

Active Controlled Study of Patients Receiving Infliximab for Treatment of Rheumatoid Arthritis of Early Onset (ASPIRE)

Purpose

The ASPIRE study[56] demonstrated that patients with early-stage RA who were treated with Remicade® and methotrexate had less progression of structural joint damage, while patients taking methotrexate alone continued to worsen.

Trial Design

ASPIRE was a randomized, double-blind, active-controlled study that enrolled 1,049 patients at 125 centers in North America and Europe. Patients were randomized to one of three study groups: Remicade® 3 mg/kg of body weight plus methotrexate; Remicade® 6 mg/kg plus methotrexate; or methotrexate alone. Remicade® was given at weeks 0, 2, 6 and every 8 weeks thereafter through week 46. The dose of methotrexate was rapidly increased in 2.5 mg increments every one to two weeks beginning with 7.5 mg per week at week 0, increasing to 15 mg per week at week 5, and stabilizing at a 20 mg per week at week 8.

---

56 Centocor, Inc. news release. Largest-ever phase III early rheumatoid study shows Remicade® plus methotrexate superior to standard of care. June 19, 2003.

The primary endpoints of the study were: (1) prevention of joint destruction; (2) prevention of disability; and (3) sustained improvement in signs and symptoms of the disease at week 54.

Clinical Results

Patients treated with all doses of Remicade® had a 44-percent overall clinical improvement, compared to a 26-percent improvement in patients treated with methotrexate only.

Sixty-six percent of patients in the Remicade® 6 mg/kg group and 62 percent of patients in the Remicade® 3 mg/kg group achieved an ACR 20 score. This compared to 54 percent in the methotrexate-only group.

More dramatic differences were observed in those patients achieving an ACR 50 and an ACR 70 response. Forty-six percent and 50 percent of patients treated with Remicade® 3 mg/kg and 6 mg/kg, respectively, achieved an ACR 50 response compared to only 32 percent of patients treated with methotrexate only. Thirty-three percent and 37 percent of patients treated with Remicade® 3 mg/kg and 6 mg/kg, respectively, achieved an ACR 70 response. This compared to only 21 percent of patients treated with methotrexate only. Additionally, 1 out of 7 Remicade®-treated patients achieved an ACR 90 response compared to only 6 percent of methotrexate-only treated patients. All results were statistically significant.

Quality of Life Measurements

Reduction in disability was measured using HAQ scores over time from week 30 to week 54. Among patients treated with Remicade® plus methotrexate, 76 percent showed a clinically meaningful improvement in functioning, versus 65 percent for patients on methotrexate alone.

THE ERA TRIAL

Drug Studied

Enbrel® (etanercept)

Study Title

Etanercept in Early Erosive Rheumatoid Arthritis (ERA) Trial

Purpose

The ERA trial compared Enbrel® and methotrexate head-on in adults with RA. Study data from this trial led to the FDA's expanded approval of Enbrel® for early-stage RA in 2000. Enbrel® is currently the only TNF blocker to be approved as a first-line agent in treating RA.

Trial Design

To qualify for the original ERA trial, participants had to be at least 18 years old with early active RA that had been diagnosed within the previous three years. They had to have at least 12 tender joints, 10 swollen joints, and either an erythrocyte sedimentation rate (ESR) greater than 28 mm/hr, a C-reactive protein (CRP) greater than 2.0 mg/dL, or morning stiffness greater than 45 minutes. Participants were also required to have never tried methotrexate therapy.

The total study population of 632 patients was randomized to one of three treatment groups: methotrexate, Enbrel® 25 mg twice weekly, or Enbrel® 10 mg twice weekly. Methotrexate dosage was gradually increased from 7.5 mg weekly to 20 mg weekly over the first eight weeks of the trial, while the Enbrel® or placebo injections were given twice weekly.

Clinical Results

Results of the original ERA trial demonstrated the safety and efficacy of Enbrel® in early, erosive RA. These results were published in 2000.[57]

Subsequent to this study, two-year data were published in 2002[58] based on 304 patients who continued into the open-label phase of the study. These 304 patients included 161 participants who had received 25 mg Enbrel® twice weekly in the original trial. It also included 143 participants who had initially been prescribed methotrexate only (average dosage 19 mg), but opted for Enbrel® treatment in the open label study. As in 2000, Enbrel® again proved safe and effective in early-stage RA.

Data from the two-year study were updated and presented at the 2002 meeting of the American College of Rheumatology.[59] Of the 161 participants who had been on Enbrel® from the study's start, 136 were available for evaluation at four years.

57 Bathon JM, Martin RW, Fleischmann RM, et al. A comparison of etanercept and methotrexate in patients with early rheumatoid arthritis. *N Engl J Med.* 2000;343:1586-1593.

58 Genovese MC, Bathon JM, Martin RW, et al. Etanercept versus methotrexate in patients with early rheumatoid arthritis: two-year radiographic and clinical outcomes. *Arthritis Rheum.* 2002;46:1443-1450.

59 Genovese MC, Martin RW, Fleischmann RM, Keystone EC, Bathon JM, Spencer-Green G. Etanercept (Enbrel®) in Early Erosive Rheumatoid Arthritis (ERA Trial): observations at 4 years. Program and abstracts of the 66th Annual Scientific Meeting of the American College of Rheumatology; October 25-29, 2002; New Orleans, Louisiana. Abstract 1419.

Among these patients, 79 percent of these patients had achieved ACR 20, 58 percent had achieved ACR 50, and 31 percent had attained ACR 70.

In addition, 27 percent of participants had no tender joints, 21 percent had no swollen joints, 23 percent had a zero HAQ score, and 73 percent had normal C-reactive protein (CRP) level.

Enbrel® also demonstrated a slowing of progressive erosions over the four-year period, as seen on x-ray. Among the 74 patients who were taking concomitant corticosteroids, 72 were able to decrease or discontinue use of the steroids by the fourth year.

Adverse Effects

At both two and four years, the incidence of serious adverse events did not increase versus those seen among participants in the original ERA trial. This applied to the number of serious infections requiring hospitalization or intravenous antibiotics as well as malignancies.

THE TEMPO TRIAL

Drug Studied

Enbrel® (etanercept)

Study Title

Trial of Etanercept and Methotrexate with Radiographic Patient Outcomes (TEMPO)

Purpose

The TEMPO trial compared the effectiveness of combined Enbrel®-methotrexate therapy against that of Enbrel® monotherapy and MTX monotherapy.

Trial Design

The TEMPO study randomized 682 patients with RA to one of three treatment arms: (1) Enbrel® only (25 mg twice weekly); (2) methotrexate only (up to 20 mg once weekly); or (3) Enbrel® 25 mg twice weekly plus methotrexate twice weekly. All participants had active RA and an inadequate response to at least one DMARD other than methotrexate. The primary radiographic endpoint was the change from baseline in the total Sharp score (TSS) at one year. Secondary radiographic endpoints included the changes in total erosions, changes in total joint space narrowing, number of eroded joints and non-progression of erosions. Health-related quality of life improvements were also evaluated using HAQ.

Clinical Results[60]

At one year, 37 percent of patients taking Enbrel®-MTX combination therapy achieved clinical remission of their RA. This compared to 18 percent of patients treated with Enbrel® alone and 14 percent of patients treated with methotrexate alone. Clinical remission was defined according to Disease Activity Score (DAS).

In addition, 80 percent of combination-therapy patients experienced no progression of joint damage. This compared to 68 percent and 57 percent, respectively, of patients treated with Enbrel® only or methotrexate only. Enbrel®-only patients experienced less progression of joint damage compared with methotrexate-only patients to a level that was statistically significant.

A substantial percentage of patients also experienced an improvement in RA symptoms. In the Enbrel®-methotrexate combination therapy group, 85 percent of patients achieved ACR 20, 69 percent achieved ACR 50 and 43 percent of patients achieved ACR 70. HAQ scores were also significantly improved among combination therapy patients. More than half (51 percent) reported an improvement of more than one point, which indicates a significant improvement in functionality.

---

60 Amgen Inc. news release. New data show many rheumatoid arthritis patients treated with Enbrel® plus methotrexate have experience clinical remission and most had no progression of joint damage. October 24, 2003.

OPEN-LABEL EXTENSION TRIAL OF ENBREL®
IN PSORIATIC ARTHRITIS

Drug Studied

Enbrel® (etanercept)

Purpose

These interim data were published for presentation at the 67th annual scientific sessions of the American College of Rheumatology held in Orlando, Florida, in October 2003. The data were drawn from an ongoing, open-label extension study to evaluate the efficacy and tolerability of Enbrel® in psoriatic arthritis patients over a longer term. Maximum treatment duration among study participants was 106 weeks.

Clinical Results[61]

Enbrel® continued to be well-tolerated and demonstrated sustained efficacy for up to 106 weeks in many patients with psoriatic arthritis. These patients experienced less joint pain, fewer swollen joints and exhibited clearer skin. Sixty-six percent of 145 patients treated with Enbrel® for at least 48 weeks achieved ACR 20, and 47 percent achieved ACR 50. Fifty-seven percent of patients also had substantial clearing of their psoriasis plaques.

---

61 Amgen Inc. news release. Long-term data support sustained efficacy, tolerability and increased vitality for psoriatic arthritis patients treated with Enbrel®. October 24, 2003.

Health-related quality of life improvements were also evaluated using HAQ. At 48 weeks, 39 percent of patients achieved a HAQ score of zero, which indicated no functional disability.

PHASE III TRIAL OF ENBREL® IN ANKYLOSING SPONDYLITIS

Drug Studied

Enbrel® (etanercept)

Purpose

These interim data were published for presentation at the 67th annual scientific sessions of the American College of Rheumatology held in Orlando, Florida, in October 2003. The data were drawn from a phase III trial of patients taking Enbrel® for ankylosing spondylitis.

Clinical Results[62]

Compared with placebo, patients taking Enbrel® generally experienced rapid and statistically significant improvement in patient-reported outcomes. These include measures of pain, overall disease activity, function and fatigue. At six months, 57 percent of Enbrel® patients achieved a 20-percent improvement in the Assessment on Ankylosing Spondylitis Response Criteria (ASAS 20).[63] This compared to 22 percent of patients in the control group. Approximately 17 percent of Enbrel® patients also reported a partial remission of their ankylosing spondylitis (as defined by an ASAS score of less than 20), compared to 4 percent of patients taking placebo.

---

62 Amgen Inc. news release. Landmark phase 3 data show ankylosing spondylitis patients experienced partial clinical remission, improved pain relieve and function. October 24, 2003.

63 The ASAS is similar to the ACR response criteria system.

APPENDIX B

Common Laboratory Tests for Arthritis

The information contained in this appendix is presented as general information. It is not intended to offer a diagnosis or personal medical advice. Always consult your physician for definitive information about your specific medical condition and laboratory test results.

ANTI-CYCLIC CITRULLINATED PEPTIDE ANTIBODY TEST

Type

Blood (serum) test

Purpose

The anti-cyclic citrullinated peptide (anti-CCP) antibody test is used to assist in the early diagnosis of rheumatoid arthritis (RA). The test is especially useful in diagnosing rheumatoid arthritis when the rheumatoid factor (RF) test is negative. (The RF test is a standard test used in arthritis diagnosis.) The anti-CCP antibody test is sometimes referred to as anti-citrullinated antibody test or simply, citrullinated antibody test.

About Anti-CCP Antibodies

The anti-cyclic citrullinated peptide antibody is an immune protein that binds to an amino acid called citrulline. The presence of these antibodies is highly specific for predicting RA, much more so than the conventional RF test.

Results and Reference Range

Results are reported as the level of anti-CCP antibodies in the blood. High levels are more likely to be associated with RA than low levels.

Interpreting Test Results

Anti-CCP antibodies have been detected in patients with RA years before the first physical symptoms of RA appear. The presence of anti-CCP antibodies is also associated with an increased risk for the more severe, erosive form of RA.

ANTI-NUCLEAR ANTIBODY TEST

Type

Blood (serum) test

Purpose

The anti-nuclear antibody (ANA) test is a diagnostic tool. A positive result by itself does not provide a definite diagnosis, but it can be useful in ruling in or ruling out autoimmune conditions such as lupus and scleroderma.

About ANA

People with certain autoimmune disorders, especially lupus, produce antibodies to the nuclei of the body's cells. A simple blood test determines the "titer," or "level" of these anti-nuclear antibodies in the blood.

Results and Reference Range

Results are reported as positive or negative. A positive result also indicates the level of ANA present in the blood.

Interpreting Test Results

A negative ANA test is considered normal, and makes a diagnosis of lupus unlikely. A positive test, especially one with a high level of ANA present is more likely to indicate an autoimmune condition and requires closer follow-up and additional evaluation. Low levels of ANA are less likely to be associated with autoimmune conditions.

Notes

While more than 95 percent of lupus patients test positive for ANA, over 5 percent of the general population have a low level of ANA in their blood without symptoms of lupus or another autoimmune condition. This is especially true for people over age 65. Thyroid disease, other inflammatory conditions and certain medications can also cause a positive ANA test.

C-REACTIVE PROTEIN TEST

Type

Blood (serum) test

Purpose

The C-reactive protein (CRP) test measures the concentration of CRP in the blood. The test is used to help confirm a diagnosis of RA or another inflammatory condition. The test is also used to monitor response to therapy.

About C-Reactive Protein

C-reactive protein is a protein that is produced by the liver during episodes of acute inflammation, such as might happen with an infection or a chronic condition like rheumatoid arthritis. Elevated levels of CRP have also been associated with an increased risk of coronary artery disease.

Results and Reference Range

Results are reported as positive or negative. A normal result finds the blood sample to be negative for CRP.

Interpreting Test Results

A positive CRP may indicate any number of inflammatory conditions, including arthritis, infection and cancer. For this reason, a positive CRP test alone is not enough to diagnose RA. It is used in combination with clinical symptoms, as well as other laboratory tests and x-ray findings.

DS-DNA ANTIBODY TEST

Type

> Blood (serum) test

Purpose

> The double-stranded (ds) DNA antibody test is used in two ways:

> - Diagnostic tool. This test is used to confirm a diagnosis of lupus after a positive anti-nuclear antibody (ANA) test.

> - Disease monitoring tool. This test is sometimes used to monitor the level of disease activity in lupus patients. An increase or decrease in the level of ds-DNA antibodies correlates with the level of disease activity.

About ds-DNA

> Antibodies to deoxyribonucleic acid (DNA) target the genetic material found in the body's cells. In the past, ds-DNA antibodies were almost always exclusive to systemic lupus erythematosus (SLE), but are now found in a small percentage of patients taking TNF blockers. Clinicians specifically look for antibodies to native, or "double-stranded," DNA in blood samples, because antibodies to single-stranded DNA are common and have no diagnostic value. About 60 percent of people with SLE produce ds-DNA antibodies, but the antibodies are rarely found in patients with other autoimmune disorders.

Results and Reference Range

Results are reported as the level of ds-DNA present in the blood. A normal result is considered less than 1.0 microgram of ds-DNA per milliliter of blood.

Interpreting Test Results

A negative test makes a diagnosis of lupus less likely. A positive test with elevated levels of ds-DNA antibodies indicates active SLE.

Note

TNF blockers may increase the level of ds-DNA antibodies in the blood, but this finding is not clinically significant, meaning that the patient does not necessarily have lupus.

ERYTHROCYTE SEDIMENTATION RATE TEST

Type

Blood (serum) test

Purpose

Erythrocyte sedimentation rate (ESR) measures how fast red blood cells (erythrocytes) cling together, fall and settle in the bottom of a specially-marked test tube over a period of one hour. This test is nonspecific; it is used to screen for any number of inflammatory conditions and diseases. The ESR test is also called a sed rate test.

About Erythrocyte Sedimentation Rate

The erythrocyte sedimentation rate allows a specific amount of the patient's blood to sit, undisturbed, in a specially marked test tube for one hour. The red blood cells separate from the plasma, which rises to the top of the tube. The red cells settle toward the bottom. Normally, red cells do not settle out in great mass. However, in certain diseases and conditions, abnormal or excess proteins cause the red cells to agglutinate. These clumps of red cells are heavier than single cells and fall faster toward the bottom of the tube. The faster the rate of settlement, the higher the column of erythrocyte sediment, and the higher the ESR.

Results and Reference Range

ESR is measured in millimeters of sedimentation per hour. The range varies between males and females. For males, the normal range is 0 to 15 mm per hour. For females, the normal range is 0 to 20 mm per hour. The normal range increases with age.

Interpreting the Test Results

In general, the higher the ESR, the greater the level of inflammation. Elevated ESR is seen in a number of conditions, ranging from anemia and pregnancy to rheumatoid arthritis and some forms of cancer. A decreased ESR can indicate sickle-cell anemia or other conditions. A definite diagnosis for a rheumatoid condition, therefore, is dependent upon a medical history, physical examination and x-rays in conjunction with other laboratory tests.

HLA-B27 TISSUE TYPING TEST

Type

Blood (serum) test

Purpose

The HLA-B27 test is a diagnostic tool. This test by itself does not provide a definite diagnosis, but it useful in distinguishing spondyloarthropathies, such as ankylosing spondylitis, psoriatic arthritis and reactive arthritis, from other types of inflammatory arthritis.

About HLA

Human leukocyte antigens (HLA) are proteins located on the surface of the white blood cells and other tissues in the body. There are two types of HLA: I and II. These main categories are further categorized into groups (Type I, groups A, B and C; and Type II, group D). Each group contains dozens of proteins, which are designated by number. HLA-B27 is one such protein. It is typically present in the blood of people with spondyloarthropathy, such as ankylosing spondylitis, psoriatic arthritis and reactive arthritis.

Results and Reference Range

Results are reported as positive or negative. A normal report finds the blood sample to be negative for HLA-B27.

Interpreting the Results

HLA-B27 is a genetic marker that is present in 90 percent of people with spondyloarthropathy, including 80 percent of people with reactive arthritis, 90 percent of people with ankylosing spondylitis, and 50 percent of people with either psoriatic arthritis or inflammatory bowel disease (IBD) that has spine involvement. (Just 10 percent of patients with psoriatic arthritis or IBD test positive for HLA-B27 when the spine isn't involved.) So, a positive HLA-B27 test may help to confirm the presence of spondyloarthropathy in patients with signs and symptoms of a spondyloarthropathic condition. However, up to 8 percent of the general population also have this genetic marker in their blood but do not develop a spondyloarthropathic illness.

RHEUMATOID FACTOR TEST

Type

Blood (serum) test

Purpose

The rheumatoid factor (RF) test is used as a diagnostic tool. The test detects the presence of an antibody called the rheumatoid factor in the blood. This test is often positive in people with rheumatoid arthritis.

The RF test is also called the RA latex test or latex fixation test. The term "latex" refers to the mechanism of the test, in which antigen-coated latex particles agglutinate with RF, if RF is present, in a sample of blood. If the test is positive for RF, the sample is titrated to measure the level of RF that is present.

About the Rheumatoid Factor

The rheumatoid factor is an antibody that binds to Fc portion of immunoglobulin G (IgG) to form a molecule known as an immune complex. (Refer to Chapter 5 for more information about immunoglobulins.) This immune complex can activate various inflammatory processes, such as those that are characteristic of rheumatoid arthritis. More than three-quarters of adults with RA test positive for the rheumatoid factor in their blood.

Results and Reference Range

Results are usually reported as positive or negative. A normal result is one that finds the blood to be negative for RF. In tests that measure the amount of RF in the blood, a level of RF less than 20 µl per milliliter of blood is considered normal.

Interpreting Test Results

A positive RF test means that you have the rheumatoid factor in your blood. RF is found in over 70 percent of adults with RA, but it is also found in people with lupus, scleroderma, hepatitis, syphilis, tuberculosis. leukemia, and a number of other diseases. RF is also found in the blood of about 5 percent of healthy adults.

WHITE BLOOD CELL COUNT

Type

Blood (serum) test. The white blood cell (WBC) count may be performed as part of a complete blood count (CBC). A CBC is a series of blood tests that provides information about the main components of blood, including red blood cells (erythrocytes), white blood cells (leukocytes) and platelets.

Purpose

The white blood cell count has two purposes:

- Screening tool. The leukocyte count indicates the absence or presence of infection or inflammation.

- Drug therapy monitoring. The leukocyte count is useful in determining whether an arthritis medication is lowering the white blood cell count, which puts you at increased risk of infections.

About White Blood Cells

White blood cells help the body fight infections and other diseases. Leukocyte is another name for white blood cell.

Results and Reference Range

Results are reported as the number of white blood cells per µl of blood. A normal result is 5,000-10,000 white blood cells per µl of blood.

Interpreting Test Results

A decreased or abnormally low leukocyte count indicates a weakened immune response, which may predispose the patient to the risk of infection. The cause of a low leukocyte count may be a viral infection or a reaction to any number of drugs, including anti-cancer medications and certain arthritis medicines. An increased or abnormally high leukocyte count signals the presence of a bacterial infection or inflammatory condition such as RA.

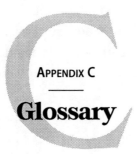

Glossary

A

ACR response criteria system. A system developed by the American College of Rheumatology (ACR) that measures clinical response to therapies used to treat rheumatoid arthritis (RA). The rating indicates the degree of improvement and is expressed as a percentage of improvement. For example, ACR 20, refers to a 20-percent improvement in the ACR's stated criteria, while ACR 50 or ACR 70 refers to a 50-percent or 70-percent improvement.

Acute. A condition characterized by rapid onset and short duration.

Acute phase reactant tests. Laboratory tests that detect an elevation in certain molecules in the blood in response to an acute condition in the body, such as infection or trauma. The infection or injury causes a rise in body temperature and white blood cell count, which peaks after several days, and usually persists after the temperature and white blood cell count normalizes. ESR and CRP tests are examples of acute phase reactant tests.

Agglutination. Clumping of cells as a result of an interaction with a specific antibody, such as what occurs between antigen-coated latex particles and rheumatoid factor during a positive rheumatoid factor test.

Amino acid. The basic building block of a protein. The structure and function of each type of protein are determined by the kinds of amino acids used to make it and how they are arranged.

Analgesic. A drug that relieves pain.

Ankylosing spondylitis. A chronic inflammatory arthritis that affects the spine and adjacent structures. It often progresses to eventual fusion or "ankylosis" of the involved joints, which causes deformity. The disease affects primarily males younger than 30, and there is a strong heredity tendency.

Antibody. A protein that is generated by the immune system. Antibodies are produced by white blood cells. They circulate in the blood seeking out and attaching to foreign proteins called antigens in order to destroy or neutralize them.

Antigen. A substance or material considered "foreign" to the body (such as a virus, bacteria or toxin). Antibodies are formed to defend against antigens.

Anti-nuclear antibodies (ANA). A marker for certain autoimmune conditions such as lupus.

Aplastic anemia. Defective development and resulting deficiency of the three types of blood cells: red blood cells, white blood cells and platelets. The condition is related to damage or destruction of the cell-generating capability of bone marrow.

Arthritis. Inflammation of a joint, usually accompanied by pain and swelling.

Autoimmune disease. Disease in which the immune system mistakenly turns on itself, targeting cells, tissues and organs of a person's own body. In rheumatoid arthritis, for example, the immune system attacks its own joints.

B

Bacteria. A large group of single-cell microorganisms that can cause infections and disease.

Bacteriophage. A virus that infects bacteria but is harmless to humans.

Baseline. In the context of a clinical trial, refers to the patient's condition at the start of the study, which serves as the criterion against which a treatment's efficacy is measured.

Biopsy. The removal of a sample of tissue for examination under a microscope to check for abnormalities or disease.

Bridge therapy. A strategy used to treat rheumatoid arthritis in which fast-acting NSAIDs or low-dose corticosteroids are prescribed for up to six months in addition to slow-acting

DMARDs. The objective is to provide relief from pain and inflammation until benefit is realized from the DMARDs.

C

Cartilage. The soft connective tissue that covers the ends of the bone where they form the joint. Cartilage is also found in the larynx, trachea, nose and ear.

Cell. The smallest living organized unit of an organization, e.g., blood cells.

Chimeric. Refers to the diverse composition of a substance.

Chronic. Persistent and long-term, such as a chronic illness.

Clinical trials. Organized tests of potential medical treatments using human volunteers. See also Phase I, Phase II, Phase III and Phase IV clinical trials.

Combination therapy. The use of two or more RA drugs at the same time in order to achieve greater benefit.

Concomitant. Concurrent; happening at the same time.

Conjunctivitis. An inflammation of the mucous membrane that covers the eyeball and eyelid. The condition is common in people with reactive arthritis.

Contraindication. A reason that makes it inadvisable to take a particular drug or undergo a certain treatment.

Controlled clinical trial. A clinical study that includes a comparison (control) group. The comparison group receives a placebo, another treatment, or no treatment at all.

Corticosteroids. A group of related substances which, like natural cortisone, reduce inflammation and irritation.

Cortisone. A natural hormone made by the adrenal gland that helps to regulate inflammation.

COX (Cyclooxygenase). An enzyme that is important in the production of prostaglandins. Prostaglandins are hormones that have important functions in many organ systems. There are two types of COX enzymes: COX-1 and COX-2.

COX-1 (Cyclooxygenase type-1). A type of enzyme that is normally present in many tissues of the body where it is active in normal cellular functions. Among the many functions of COX-1 enzymes are protection of the stomach lining and maintenance of blood flow to the kidneys.

COX-2 (Cyclooxygenase type-2). A type of enzyme that is produced in large amounts during inflammation. COX-2 contributes to the pain and swelling associated with arthritis.

COX-2 inhibitors. A class of arthritis drugs (Celebrex®, Vioxx® and Bextra®) used to relieve pain and inflammation. These drugs selectively block the "harmful" COX-2 enzymes, and are generally considered to be more protective of the stomach than traditional NSAIDs, which block both COX-1 and COX-2 enzymes.

C-reactive protein (CRP). A protein found in the blood of people with inflammatory conditions, such as rheumatoid arthritis.

Crohn's disease. A chronic inflammatory bowel disease.

Cross-over study. Refers to a clinical study where patients taking placebo or a standard treatment are permitted to "cross over" into the experimental treatment group so that they may attempt to get benefit from the treatment under investigation.

Cyclic citrullinated peptide (CCP). A protein that is found in the blood. Antibodies to this peptide are a marker for cases of early rheumatoid arthritis that may develop into severe, erosive RA.

Cytokine. A protein produced by white blood cells that acts as a chemical messenger between cells. The result of cytokine activity is to either stimulate or inhibit the activity of various cells of the immune system.

D

Demyelinating disorders. Diseases that involve the destruction or removal of the protective myelin sheath from the nerves. Multiple sclerosis is an example of a demyelinating disease.

Disease Activity Score (DAS). A tool used to measure the extent of disease activity in RA. The score is calculated by the number of tender and swollen joints in combination with erythrocyte sedimentation rate (ESR).

Distal. A term used to describe the part of the body farthest from the trunk. For example, the toes are distal to the ankle.

DMARDs. Disease-modifying, anti-rheumatic drugs. Slow-acting or second-line agents used to treat rheumatoid arthritis to slow the progression of the disease. DMARDs are also sometimes called slow-acting anti-rheumatic drugs.

Double-blind. A type of clinical trial in which neither the participants nor the researchers know whether the placebo treatment or active treatment is being administered to a given patient. The purpose of double-blind studies is to eliminate bias in evaluating the efficacy of a treatment.

E

Efficacy. Effectiveness; the term is often used to describe the effectiveness of a medical treatment.

Endpoint. Termination point of a clinical trial, based on the attainment of a clinical status or the passage of a specified period of time.

Enthesitis. Inflammation of an enthesis. An enthesis is the site where a ligament or tendon attaches to a bone.

Enzyme. A protein that causes chemical reactions in living tissue.

Erosion. Small hole in the cartilage or bone resulting from inflammation.

Erythrocyte. Red blood cell.

Erythrocyte sedimentation rate (ESR). Commonly known as "sed rate." It is the rate at which red blood cells settle out in a tube of unclotted blood. Elevated ESR rates are not specific to any disease, but indicate inflammation. Certain noninflammatory conditions, such as pregnancy, are also associated with an elevated ESR.

Extension trial. Extension of a clinical trial beyond its original endpoint.

F

Functional Assessment of Chronic Illness Therapy (FACIT). A collection of questionnaires designed to measure health-related, quality of life issues in people with chronic illness, such as rheumatoid arthritis.

Fibromyalgia. A chronic condition characterized by muscle pain and fatigue. The cause is unknown but may be related to a problem with sleep. There is no blood test to confirm the diagnosis, and all laboratory and x-rays are usually normal.

Food and Drug Administration (FDA). The federal agency that oversees the regulation of food, pharmaceuticals and medical devices in the United States.

Fusion protein. A protein that is produced by splicing strands of genetically engineered DNA.

G

Gout. A type of arthritis caused by high levels of uric acid in the blood. Diet is implicated in gout because uric acid levels are increased by ingesting food with high purine content.

H

Health Assessment Questionnaire (HAQ). A clinical tool used to assess quality of life in patients with RA. It measures the degree of difficulty that a patient has in accomplishing everyday activities of daily living.

Human leukocyte antigens (HLA). Proteins that are located on the surface of cells. Certain HLAs are markers for arthritic conditions, e.g., HLA-B27 in ankylosing spondylitis and reactive arthritis, and HLA-DR4 in rheumatoid arthritis.

I

IgG1. The major immunoglobulin that circulates in the blood. IgG1 is able to enter other cellular structures, where it binds with antigens and facilitates their removal by other cells in the immune system. TNF antagonists are based on the IgG1 immunoglobulin.

Immune response. The activation of the immune system against foreign substances (antigens).

Immune system. The organs and cells that defend the body against infection and disease.

Immunocompromised. Having a weakened immune system, a condition that can be caused by certain diseases or treatments.

Immunoglobulin (Ig). A protein that acts as an antibody.

Immunology. The study of the body's immune system.

Immunosuppression. Suppression of the body's immune system and its ability to fight infections or disease. Certain diseases, such as AIDS and lymphoma, and treatments, such as MTX and TNF antagonists, cause immunosuppression.

Immunotherapy. Treatment that is intended to stimulate or restore the ability of the immune system to fight infection and disease.

Inflammation. A complex immune response in which cells and chemicals associated with the immune system go to the site of an infection, injury or damage. The result is marked by four signs: redness, warmth, swelling and pain.

J

Juvenile chronic arthritis (JCA). A form of rheumatoid arthritis with onset before age 16. Also called juvenile arthritis or juvenile rheumatoid arthritis.

K

Kilodalton. A measure of molecular mass.

L

Leukocyte. A white blood cell; used to ward off infection.

Leukopenia. An abnormal drop in the number of white blood cells to fewer than 4,000 cells per cubic millimeter. The condition may be caused by an adverse drug reaction or disease.

Lupus. See SLE.

Lymphocyte. A type of white blood cell involved in inflammation and fighting infection.

M

Macrophage. A type of white blood cell that surrounds and kills microorganisms, removes dead cells, and stimulates the action of other immune system cells.

Malignancy. A cancerous tumor that can invade and destroy nearby tissue, and spread to other parts of the body.

Marker. A diagnostic indication that a certain disease may develop.

Methotrexate (MTX). A slow-acting DMARD that is used in low doses to treat inflammatory disorders, including rheumatoid arthritis, psoriatic arthritis and ankylosing spondylitis. MTX is also used in very high doses to treat certain cancers.

Milligram (mg). A measure of weight, equal to about 1/28,000th of an ounce.

Monoclonal antibodies (mAb). Laboratory-produced substances that can locate and bind to specific cells, such as TNF-α.

Monotherapy. Use of a single medication to treat a disease or medical condition.

Morbidity. A disease or the incidence of disease within a population. Morbidity can also refer to adverse effects caused by a treatment.

Multi-center study. A clinical trial that is carried out at more than one medical institution.

Multiple sclerosis (MS). A disorder of the central nervous system marked by weakness, numbness, a loss of muscle coordination, and problems with vision, speech, and bladder control. Multiple sclerosis is thought to be an autoimmune disease in which the body's immune system destroys myelin. Myelin is a substance that contains both protein and fat (lipid), serving as a nerve insulator and helping in the transmission of nerve signals.

Musculoskeletal. Involving the tissues of the skeletal system, including muscles, bones, cartilage, tendons and ligaments.

N

National Institutes of Health (NIH). A U.S. government-sponsored biomedical research agency that conducts its own research and supports the research of scientists in universities, medical schools, hospitals, and research institutions around the country.

Necrosis. Refers to the death of living tissue.

Nodule. A small solid mass of tissue that can be felt in the skin. In people with rheumatoid arthritis, these nodules usually occur in pressure points of the body, most commonly, the elbows.

NSAIDs. Non-steroidal anti-inflammatory drugs. A category of drugs commonly prescribed to treat inflammation and pain associated with arthritis and other musculoskeletal conditions.

Nucleus. The command center within a living cell. The nucleus contains the genetic codes (in chromosomes) for maintaining cellular processes and for issuing commands for cell growth and reproduction.

O

Off-label. Use of a drug for other than an FDA-approved application.

Open label trial. Refers to a clinical trial in which both the participants and researchers know what treatment the participant is taking and at what dose, as opposed to a blind trial in which participants and/or researchers do not know what therapy the patient is undergoing.

Osteoarthritis (OA). The most common form of arthritis. In OA, the cartilage (the protective cushion in joints), wears down, causing pain and inflammation. Weight-bearing joints, such as the knees and hips, as well as the hands, are the most common sites of involvement.

P

Pancytopenia. A condition characterized by a decrease in all types of blood cells.

Pathology. Study of the essential nature of diseases and the structural and functional changes caused by it. Or, structural and functional deviations from the normal, healthy state that characterize a particular disease.

Peptide. A group of amino acids that are linked together. Multiple peptides form proteins, which are the basic building blocks of the body.

Phase I trial. A clinical study that evaluates the safety, appropriate dosage levels, and general response to a new treatment. Because little is known about the possible risks and benefits of the treatments being tested, phase I trials usually include only a small number of patients who have not been helped by other treatments.

Phase II trial. A clinical study to test whether a new treatment has benefit in a certain disease process or for a specific medical condition.

Phase III trial. A clinical study to compare the results of a new treatment against a standard treatment or placebo.

Phase IV trial. A clinical study that evaluates "post-marketing" side effects in a larger population that may not have been apparent in Phase III studies. Phase IV trials take place after a treatment has been approved by the FDA and made available to the general population.

Placebo. An inactive substance that looks the same and is administered in the same way as a drug in a clinical trial, but has no pharmacologic action against a patient's illness or complaint. In a clinical trial, placebo treatment given to the control group allows the effects of the experimental treatment to be measured.

Platelet. The component of blood responsible for clotting.

Polyarticular. Refers to the involvement of many joints, such as polyarticular juvenile chronic arthritis.

Post-marketing. A term used to describe events that occur after a drug has been approved by the FDA for commercial marketing.

Prognosis. The probable outcome of a disease.

Prostaglandins. Substances that have important functions in many organ systems, including the production of mucous to protect the stomach lining.

Protein. A large molecule composed of amino acids, and an essential component of body tissue (see also peptide).

Proximal. A term used to describe the part of the body closest to the trunk. For example, the wrist is proximal to the fingers.

Psoriatic arthritis. A type of inflammatory arthritis that is associated with psoriasis, a chronic skin and nail disease.

Pyrimidine. An enzyme associated with joint inflammation.

R

Randomized clinical trial. A study in which the participants are assigned randomly to different treatment groups. Random assignment ensures that the treatment groups will be similar, which allows an unbiased evaluation of the treatments.

Raynaud's phenomenon. A disorder of the small blood vessels of the extremities that causes reduced blood flow. In response to cold or anxiety, these vessels go into spasms, causing pain, the sensations of burning and tingling, and color changes, typically from blue to white to red.

Reactive arthritis. Arthritis resulting from infection elsewhere in the body; i.e., there is no infection in the joint. This type of arthritis is characterized by joint inflammation, conjunctivitis, and urethritis, with or without other features of spondyloarthropathy. The most common type is HLA B27-related and may follow certain types of bowel or genitourinary infection. Reactive arthritis was formerly called Reiter's syndrome.

Receptor. A molecule inside or on the surface of a cell that binds to a specific substance and causes a specific physiologic effect in the cell.

Recombinant. Refers to a substance made through genetic engineering, which is also called "gene splicing" or "recombinant DNA technology." By putting human genes into the genetic material of living cells, these microorganisms can be turned into "factories" to make human proteins for medical uses.

Reiter's syndrome. See reactive arthritis.

Rheumatic diseases. A group of conditions characterized by inflammation or pain in the muscles, joints, and fibrous tissue. Rheumatic diseases or disorders can be related to autoimmunity or other causes.

Rheumatoid arthritis (RA). A type of inflammatory arthritis involving the hands, feet and other joints. RA involves prolonged morning joint stiffness that lessens as the day goes on, with involvement of at least four joints. It most commonly afflicts women between the ages of 30 and 60.

Rheumatoid factor (RF). A diagnostic marker for rheumatoid arthritis. About 75 percent of people with RA have RF in their blood. RF is also found in about 5 percent of healthy people.

Rheumatologist. A specialist who treats rheumatic illnesses.

Rheumatology. A subspecialty of internal medicine that involves the non-surgical evaluation and treatment of the rheumatic diseases and conditions.

S

Sacroiliac joints. Lower back joints; specifically the two joints located between the sacrum (the five fused vertebrae in the lower spine) and the ilium (bones of the pelvis).

Sciatica. Pain that runs along the course of a sciatic nerve, especially in the back of the thigh and down the leg.

Sclerodactyly. The hard, shiny appearance of fingers caused by excess connective tissue buildup. It is a common feature of scleroderma.

Scleroderma. A chronic illness characterized by hardening and thickening of the skin. Scleroderma can be localized (morphea) or it can affect the entire body (systemic).

Screening. Checking for disease when there are no symptoms.

Sed rate. See ESR.

Sepsis. Often referred to as a "bloodstream infection" that can be life-threatening. Sepsis involves the presence of bacteria or other infectious organisms in the blood (septicemia) or in other body tissues. Sepsis may be associated with clinical symptoms of systemic illness, such as fever, chills, low blood pressure, and diminished mental alertness.

Seronegative. Negative for the presence of a specific antibody, such as the rheumatoid factor, in the serum of blood.

Seropositive. Positive for the presence of a specific antibody, such as the rheumatoid factor, in the serum of blood.

Serum. The clear liquid that can be separated from clotted blood. Serum is different than plasma, which is the liquid portion of normal unclotted blood that contains red blood cells, white blood cells and platelets.

Sharp score. A method for evaluating changes in total joint damage by assessing the number of bone erosions and the amount of joint space narrowing as seen on x-ray.

Single-blind. Refers to a clinical trial in which the participants do not know if they are getting the placebo or the active substance. However, the physicians and/or researchers do know which substance the participants have been given.

Sjögren's syndrome. An autoimmune condition characterized by dry mouth, eyes, and other mucous membranes. Arthritis may also be present. The symptoms of this disorder affect primarily women over the age of 40. It may occur in association with other rheumatic diseases.

Spondylitis. Inflammation of the spine. The term is sometimes confused with spondylosis, which is a noninflammatory degenerative disease of the spine.

Spondyloarthropathy. A disease that affects the joints of the spine, such as ankylosing spondylitis, psoriatic arthritis, reactive arthritis and inflammatory bowel disease.

Statistical significance. Demonstration, through statistical methods, that a result obtained in a clinical trial is due to the treatment being studied, because the probability of obtaining such a result by chance alone is relatively low.

Stevens-Johnson syndrome. A type of hypersensitivity (allergic) reaction that occurs in response to medications, infection or illness. The condition causes severe swelling and destruction of the skin and mucous membranes, and can be life-threatening.

Syndrome. A group, or complex, of signs and symptoms that when occur together, suggest a particular disease. Sjögren's syndrome is an example.

Synovial fluid. The fluid that lubricates joints and provides nutrients to the cartilage.

Systemic. Occurring throughout the body as a whole, as opposed to affecting a localized site or on a limited scope.

Systemic lupus erythematosus (SLE). A condition where the immune system is overactive, causing inflammation in the joints, skin and organs such as the kidneys and lungs. SLE is one of four types of lupus; two other forms affect primarily the skin; the fourth is induced by certain medications.

T

T cell. A type of white blood cell that plays a central role in inflammation.

Titer. The minimum volume of a substance necessary to allow a measurement to be made.

TNF blockers. A category of drug that inhibits the effect of TNF-alpha and has shown benefit in certain types of arthritis and autoimmune diseases. Also called TNF antagonists.

Toxicity. A condition that results from exposure to a substance, e.g., a drug, that may not cause adverse effects in smaller amounts or during short-term use.

Treatment arm. In the context of a clinical trial, another term for a treatment group.

Tuberculosis. An infectious disease that usually attacks the lungs, but can attack almost any of the body's organ systems.

Tumor Necrosis Factor-alpha (TNF-α). A pro-inflammatory cytokine that is present in large quantities in people with RA.

Tumor Necrosis Factor-beta (TNF-β). Another type of pro-inflammatory cytokine that plays a role (in conjunction with TNF-α) in juvenile chronic arthritis.

U

Uveitis. Inflammation of the inner eye. The condition is common in people with spondyloarthropathies.

V

Vaccine. A substance or group of substances injected in an attempt to cause the immune system to respond to a specific antigen or microorganism in order to build immunity against it.

Vasculitis. Inflammation of blood vessels caused by an immune reaction in the vessel walls. Vasculitis can occur in several autoimmune diseases, including RA, lupus and scleroderma.

Virus. A microorganism that can infect cells and cause disease.

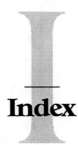

Index

Enbrel® *cont'd.*

   safety profile

      in adults, 100-05

      in children, 106

   and sciatica, 182

   and sepsis, 146

   side effects, 91-92, 101, 145-46, 162-63, 172-73

   and surgery, 162-63

   talking with your physician about, 147-52

   and tuberculosis, 85, 100, 104, 143, 146

   traveling with, 161, 179

   use of other medications with, 107, 171

   and vaccinations, 107, 150, 164-65, 175-76

Enliven® Program, 152, 157

ERA Trial, 200-02

Erythrocyte Sedimentation Rate (ESR)

   and Disease Activity Score (DAS), 189, 230

   defined, 216, 232

   test, 132, 188-89, 200, 216-17

   use in diagnosing ankylosing spondylitis, 16

   use in diagnosing rheumatoid arthritis, 11

Etanercept (see Enbrel®)

Etodolac (see Lodine®)

Ewing, Julie, 109

F

Fibromyalgia, 33-34

FluMist™ Intranasal Influenza Virus Vaccine, 107, 120, 128, 164, 175

Folinic Acid (leucovorin), 42

Food and Drug Administration Arthritis Advisory Committee, 62, 87-88, 105, 117

Functional Assessment of Chronic Illness Therapy (FACIT), 190, 195

G

Garrett, Connie, 142

Glucosamine, 8

Gold Sodium Thiomalate (see Myochrysine®)

Gold Therapy, 39, 95, 132

Gordon, Rose, 150

Gout, 22-24

H

Health Assessment Questionnaire (HAQ), 37, 190, **199**, 202, 203, 204, 206, 233

Heart Attack

   and COX-2 inhibitors, 51-52, 53

Heart Failure (see Congestive Heart Failure)

Hollingsworth, Joy, 82

Holt, Susan, 95

Honeywell, Bob, 3, 183

Human Leukocyte Antigens (HLA), 218, 233

Humira™ (see also TNF Blockers)

   administration, 123, 148, 153-54, 156-59, 177

   adverse effects (see also side effects), 92, 124, 145-46

   and anti-nuclear antibody (ANA) development, 125

   ARMADA trial, 194

   and autoantibody development, 85-86, 125

   at a glance, 123

Humira™ *cont'd.*

  traveling with, 161, 179

  and tuberculosis, 85, 124, 127, 143, 146

  use of other medications with, 128, 171

  and vaccinations, 119, 150, 164-65, 175-76

HLA-B27

  defined, 218, 233

  presence in ankylosing spondylitis, 17, 218

  presence in IBD-associated arthritis, 21

  presence in psoriatic arthritis, 18, 218

  presence in reactive arthritis, 20, 218, 240

  presence in spondyloarthropathy, 14, 218

  test, 218-219

Hydrocodone, 171

Hydroxychloroquine Sulfate (see Plaquenil®)

I

Ibuprofen (e.g., Advil®, Motrin®), 8, 36, 40, 51

IgG, IgG1, 78-79, 81, 98, 111, 123, 182, 220, 233

IL-1 (see Interleukins)

Immunex Corporation, xi, xii

Immunoglobulins, 78-79, 220

Imuran® (azathioprine), 21, 25, 39, 132

Infections

  and Arava®, 61

  and Enbrel®, 83-84, 100, 104, 106, 162, 202

  and Humira™, 83-84, 124, 127-28, 162, 196

Infections *cont'd.*

  and Kineret®, 68

  and methotrexate, 43

  and Remicade®, 83-84, 113, 114, 118-19, 162

  and TNF blockers, 83-84, 92, 133, 143, 145-46, 148, 162, 163, 165, 171, 172, 174, 176

Inflammatory Bowel Disease

  associated with arthritis, 20-22

  diagnosis, 21

  and HLA-B27, 21

  symptoms, 21, 22

  treatment, 21, 22

Infliximab (see Remicade®)

Influenza Virus Vaccine, intranasal (see FluMist™)

Injectable Gold (see Myochrysine®)

Interleukins, xi, 66, 72, 182

Isaacs, Demetria, 181, 183

J

Juvenile Chronic Arthritis (JCA)

  defined, 12-13, 234, 239

  and Enbrel®, 96, 97, 99, 106, 136, 143, 174

  and tumor necrosis factor, 75, 245

  types of, 13-14

K

Karp, David, M.D., Ph.D., vii

Kineret®

  contraindications, 67

  description and use, 50, 66

  dosage and regimen, 66-67

  drug interactions, 68

  how it works, 66

Pregnancy Risk Category, 89

Probenecid (see Benemid®)

Proximal Interphalangeal (PIP) Joints, 10, 11

Pruett, Angie, 127, 149

Psoriatic Arthritis

defined, 17

diagnosing, 18

and Enbrel®, 3, 76, 95, 96, 97, 99, 100, 104, 107, 136, 140, 141, 143, 149, 205

and HLA-B27, 18, 218

and HLA-B27 test, 18, 218

and Humira™, 174

and rheumatoid factor (RF), 18

signs and symptoms, 14, 17

treatment options, 18

and trials of Enbrel®, 205

and tumor necrosis factor, 75, 135, 172

types of, 18-19

Q

Questran® (cholestyramine), 61, 64, 65

R

Raynaud's Phenomenon, 31, 240

Reactive Arthritis

and conjunctivitis, 19

defined, 15, 19, 240

genitourinary involvement, 19

and HLA-B27, 20, 218, 233

and HLA-B27 test, 20, 218

and the rheumatoid factor (RF), 19

signs and symptoms, 19

treatment, 20

Receptors (p55, p75, TNF-α), 73, 111, 123

Recombinant Technology, 67, 78, 79, 98, 111, 123, 241

Reiter's Syndrome (see Reactive Arthritis)

Relafen® (nabumetone), 36

Remicade® (see also TNF Blockers)

administration, 110, 111, 112, 153-54, 177

adverse effects (see also side effects), 92, 114-119, 145-46

anti-nuclear antibody (ANA) development, 85-86, 115

ASPIRE trial, 197-98

at a glance, 111

and autoantibody development, 115

and blood disorders, 86

and cancer (malignancy), 86-87, 93, 115-16

and cardiopulmonary events, 90-91

and central nervous system disorders, 89, 116, 164

clinical trial results, 197-98

combination therapy with methotrexate, 112

compared with other TNF blockers, 120, 141, 143-46

composition, 80-81, 111, 143

and congestive heart failure, 90-91, 113, 116-17

contraindications, 113-14, 143

cost, 93, 111, 137-39, 146, 151

and Crohn's disease, 76, 110

and demyelinating disorders, 116, 146

description and use, 76, 112, 143, 174

and diabetes, 113, 163

Printed in the United States
118328LV00003B/275/A